CHRONIC PAIN
MY JOURNEY

DON S HUNTER

Chronic Pain: My Journey
Copyright © 2023 by Don S Hunter

All rights reserved. No part of this publication may be reproduced, distributed, or transmitted in any form or by any means, including photocopying, recording, or other electronic or mechanical methods, without the prior written permission of the author, except in the case of brief quotations embodied in critical reviews and certain other non-commercial uses permitted by copyright law.

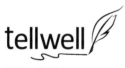

Tellwell Talent
www.tellwell.ca

ISBN
978-0-2288-8591-7 (Hardcover)
978-0-2288-8592-4 (Paperback)
978-0-2288-8590-0 (eBook)

*We may not be able to eliminate pain, but
we can reduce our suffering.*

This is a wise book. Don Hunter draws you into his story effortlessly, describing a remarkably full life lived with chronic pain. He writes about his experience of pain realistically and compassionately, but with no hint of self-pity. At the same time, this book contains relevant and accurate information about the complex nature of chronic pain and its treatment. Using his perspective as a health care professional combined with his lived experience of pain, Mr. Hunter has provided us with a guide to taking care of oneself, not just by seeking medical care, but also by practicing self care of one's mind, body and spirit. Although everyone's journey with chronic pain is unique, this book is a road map created by a kind and brave fellow traveler.

Jan Carstoniu MD FRCPC

Through an entertaining narrative weave, Don reveals deft insight into how childhood trauma and his evolution as a therapist echo a thought after a head injury that triggered fears that he would die; "What will be will be."

However, his journey manifests a life well lived, through immeasurable chronic pain, showing us all that the strength of the human spirit is stronger than anything that can happen to it.

Phyllis Ellis, award winning filmmaker,
Olympian and partner in chronic pain.

TABLE OF CONTENTS

Dedication ix
Preface xi
Introduction xiii
Chapter 1:   My Early Life 1
Chapter 2:   The Middle Years and Adolescence 9
Chapter 3:   What to Do 27
Chapter 4:   Career and Family 35
Chapter 5:   The Pain Arrives 45
Chapter 6:   Into the Abyss 61
Chapter 7:   Climbing Out 75
Chapter 8:   Routines and Rituals 81
Chapter 9:   Creating Safe Quiet Space 89
Chapter 10: Easier Said than Done 101
Chapter 11: Semi-Retirement 115
Acknowledgements 119
Bibliography 121
Appendix A 125
About the Author 127

DEDICATION

To Annie, Ben and Luc who have been with me through this journey. Thank you for your constant love and compassion, as I know I would not be here without you!

PREFACE

January 1997, One Night.

Whatever I was dreaming is gone in a flash as a piercing blade of pain repeatedly penetrates my right temple, making me wince. My right hand instinctively places pressure on my temple, as I groggily remove the blackout mask with my left. I squint to see the time.

Already 3:30 a.m.

Repeated stabs of pain.

I curse, pull myself up and begin my deep breathing and chanting exercises. As I reach for my medication pouch, I acknowledge that my first thought is always *Just take it all and fucking end it.* Of course, I refocus on my breath and speak the words of the chant:

"There is no pain or cause in pain or cease in pain or noble path to lead from pain…"

I search my pouch for the Gravol and another Triazolam; I can't put a new Fentanyl patch on for another twenty-four hours, so I turn the heating pad on and place it over the patch to deliver whatever is left quickly. The pain spreads behind my eyes and across both temples like a forest fire, taking my attention. I get two Gravol and the Triazolam down and re-focus.

"So know that the Bodhisattva holding to nothing whatever but dwelling in Prajna wisdom is freed of delusive hindrance, rid of the fear bred by it and comes to clearest Nirvana…"

I pray to the Bodhisattvas to be with me and to guide me.
I pray to my guardian angels to dull the pain.
I pray to God to take my soul before I wake.
Surely one of them will show compassion?
I slowly get out of bed, grab an ice pack from the freezer and trudge back to the bedroom. I slide down on one of my four pillows and ice my right temple. The heat goes back on my right bicep on top of the 100mcg patch. My eyes wet with tears, I remind myself that crying can be a good release. This morning, it only increases the pain. I continue my positive self-talk, prayers and chants, waiting for the stabbing to decrease.
"You okay?"
Annie's soft voice seems far away.
"Yeh, I'm fine."
I drift off to a dream left unfinished knowing the alarm will blast into my consciousness in less than an hour, time to get ready for work. I turn the heating pad off, which I know I should not have left on, and rise slowly, sit for a few moments on the edge of the bed before I rise to stand, if I rise too quickly, I see the stars in front of my eyes and the pain between my temples increases. This was a good night because I got about four hours sleep, too many nights I get much less!

INTRODUCTION

This manuscript, a mix of journaling and academic research, has been in the works for over twenty years. I have extensively researched how to manage chronic pain and practiced virtually all of the techniques: various forms of meditation, prayer, chanting, a vast array of over-the-counter and prescription medications, cognitive behavioural therapy, homeopathy, surgery, nerve blocks, Botox injections, chiropractic adjustments, narrative therapy, hypnotherapy, compassion-focused therapy, eye movement desensitization and reprocessing therapy, neurolinguistic programming techniques, and emotion-focused therapy. I consistently became engrossed in each of these areas, learning and practicing the wide variety of skills and techniques they offer. In developing this manuscript, I weighed the pros and cons of focusing strictly on managing chronic pain or focusing on my personal struggle living with daily chronic pain. As I wrote about a typical night's events, I realized that the experience of putting it down on paper provided some relief and, strangely, a sense of purpose. However, it is often difficult to predict either the quality or duration of pain and some of my writing occurs when the pain is intense and other parts when the pain has eased somewhat. My experiences are presented as they occurred in my life, my apologies if some portions seem randomly placed.

It became clear that my experiences before the pain came into my life, my personal struggle with the pain and its impact on my personal and professional life are all connected and intertwined. Because of this realization, it simply made sense to write about my experiences that captured the whole picture without getting lost in theories. I am hopeful that readers who are living with pain will find resonance in my struggles. I am also hopeful that professionals involved with clients who are struggling with pain will connect with the strategies and techniques presented. If you live with pain, I cannot advise you to use techniques that I have used, without consulting with your own team of professionals – I will present what helped and did not help – for me.

The trajectory of my life was clear until the pain arrived in November 1981. Getting to sleep and staying asleep became increasingly difficult, so for about the next ten years I self-medicated with a combination of decongestants and Tylenol 3s to dull the pain so I could get to sleep. By 1990, I was up to twelve Tylenol 3s a day just to get through work and not "give in" to the pain.

I consulted a pain specialist and spent the next ten years experimenting with different combinations of narcotics. I was on daily Fentanyl patches and a cocktail of other narcotics by 1997 for what one pain specialist called "breakthrough pain." I then began taking a powerful sedative to allow me to get more than four hours of continuous sleep. Sound, restful sleep? No.

My determination to work, provide for my family and become the best therapist I could be has been my greatest ally in this battle. I battled the pain, frustration, worry, fear, sadness, helplessness, anger and hopelessness every day. It begins with an awareness of pain, leading to worry and fear of how bad it will get. I use various techniques to eliminate or dull the pain, but they don't provide significant relief. This triggers the frustration and anger, which makes the pain worse, leading to the helplessness and hopelessness. Most of these medications and treatments were helpful in winning "skirmishes" here and there, but I lost every major battle until 2018 when I finally surrendered and accepted the pain as a continuous presence in my life. A very annoying partner who I am stuck with!

My intention was to simply describe my life with chronic daily pain and the suffering that so often accompanies it—but pain does not exist independent of everyone around you. Pain impacts family, friends, colleagues and those involved in providing treatment. Each person has their own unique relationship with the pain. However, the actual physical relationship with the pain is only experienced by one person. I was once free of chronic pain, and various aspects of my story, experiences with pain and loss, relationships with family, social and academic experiences, provided the foundation for how I would manage what was to come.

CHAPTER 1

MY EARLY LIFE

Born in 1951, I spent the first five years of my life at 15 Exeter Street in the west end of Toronto (around St. Clair Avenue and Caledonia Road) in a three-story semi-detached house at the end of the street. Right beside our house was a large field of enormous hydro towers and a set of cold, rusted, iron train tracks about 100 yards from our house. I vividly remember the sound of the trains at night—the relentless chugging and the muffled whistle as the trains passed. I still find the sound of trains relaxing.

My childhood was spent running through the field with friends, trying to climb the hydro towers and putting an ear on the rail of the train tracks to see if we could judge how long before a train came. The rails on the tracks were always hot in the summer and ice cold in the winter, and the pungent smell of creosote that soaked the wooden railway ties often stung my nostrils.

"I can feel it's coming!" we would yell to each other. "Get off the tracks—it's coming soon!"

We would stand about fifteen feet from the tracks, adrenalin pumping, listening for the sound of the steam engine and hearing that chugging just before we could see the engine coming around the bend. We waved at the conductor and counted the rusty container cars—some closed, some loaded with brand new cars and trucks, others with open slats so the animals (usually cows or horses) could breathe. Once we could see the end of the train approaching, we would take a few steps closer so we could see the conductor on the final car—the red caboose—and we would wave frantically. He would always return the wave.

Each morning, my mom would gently rub my shoulder.

"Time to get up, Donnie."

The yeasty aroma of baked bread floated in through the window from the Weston Bakery only a few blocks away. The slaughterhouse on St. Clair was there, too, but I preferred the smell of the bakery!

I have early memories of experiences I had with both my mother and my paternal grandmother (nana) that I believe laid the foundation for the growth and development of my ability to be empathic. The seeds of compassion were planted early, as they often are. I have a vivid memory of being three or four and standing in the TV room in our home where we would watch *Captain Kangaroo* each morning. There was an old, overstuffed flowered couch and two overstuffed armchairs covered with a dark-coloured rose pattern, and an old twenty-four-inch black and white television that crackled with static every time it was turned on. There were three heavy, flowered drapes that, when drawn together, ran the full length across the room from floor to ceiling, which effectively separated the TV room from the sitting room and dining area. The smell of old wax rose up from the dark, hardwood floors that creaked when the adults walked through. There was also the faint odour of mothballs that escaped from the closets and that musty smell that crept up from the cold, dark, damp basement. I had many nightmares about what lived in the crawl space at the back of the basement!

From the living room, I was able to peek through the drapes to watch whatever was going on in the other room. One particular mid-morning when I was about three, the sun was shining through the high windows in the TV room. The drapes were drawn, but through the crack in the drapes, Mom, Nana and a woman I recognized as a neighbour were seated on an old love seat, facing the drapes. They were consoling the woman, who was hunched over, hands in her lap crying hysterically. I watched as my mom and Nana worked hard to try to console her. Nana handed her tissues and rubbed her back and shoulders.

"It's going to be okay," Nana said. "Bill is with God now."

The woman's head flew back as she screamed, "No, I need him here with me!"

Mom was crouched down at the woman's knees, and she softly said, "It will be okay, honey, Bill's not in pain anymore."

"I need him more than God! The children need him more than God!" the woman said. "How can I do this without Bill? I need to be with him!" she screamed.

Mom wrapped her arms around the woman's knees and said, "Bill's gone, honey, and it is so painful. But he would want you to be strong and take care of yourself and the kids."

As Mom repeated this phrase and Nana continued to rub the woman's shoulders, the intensity of her emotion seemed to ease. Mom and Nana were so calm, validating and reassuring. In that moment, the seeds of compassion were planted.

I teared up. I was confused about where Bill went, but it was clear he would not be coming back. The woman eventually regained some composure. I recall feeling upset. I wanted to turn away and watch the television, but I was drawn to the drama unfolding in the other room; I couldn't stop listening. Now I realize that I was witnessing the core components of empathy and compassion being demonstrated by the two most important people in my life.

The next experience that had a significant impact on me during my earliest years was watching *The Wizard of Oz* every year! My dad was a salesman and was often on the road. My older brother Brad, my mom, Nana and Grandpa would make hot chocolate and shortbread cookies for the event. Snuggling with my nana in one of the overstuffed, flowered armchairs, I would always hide my face in her arms when the wicked witch confronted Dorothy. Fear rose in my chest as I waited for the terrifying flying monkeys to arrive. When Dorothy sang *Somewhere Over the Rainbow*, my nana would say, "That means all your dreams can come true!"

She was the foundation of my hopeful, optimistic self. My nana was a tiny Irish woman with grey, curly hair, glasses, and a soft, warm smile. And she gave the best hugs! My nana's optimism stayed with me and helped me through many difficult and painful times. She was born and raised in Dublin, Ireland, and my grandfather was born and raised in Edinburgh, Scotland.

Although my nana was so very kind and patient, my grandpa had little patience and a bit of a temper, both of which he passed on to my dad. Grandpa was a short, gruff Scotsman who served in the First World War, lost his hearing, and refused to show any vulnerability. Everyone had to raise their voice and repeat things for Grandpa to hear them. The response would often begin with, "I heard you, for Pete's sake. You don't have to yell!" At some point along the way, Grandpa finally got a hearing aid, but it was quite a cumbersome thing—a three-inch square device that clipped to the front of his shirt that had a long twisted white cord running up to his left ear. He was always playing with the volume and tapping the device because it wasn't working. We could often hear the loud whistle from the earpiece, which did not seem to fit properly.

My mom was much more patient. She also loved to laugh and almost always responded positively to my joking and goofing around. She used to sing *Que Sera Sera* to us at night and on long trips in the car.

"What does that mean?" I asked once.

She looked at me and said, "That means, what will be, will be, Donnie."

I believe this was a core belief that had been passed down from generation to generation. My dad was different, as he seemed to find my humour childish and somewhat aggravating until my later adolescence, when he was able to relax more and enjoy family relationships.

CHRONIC PAIN: MY JOURNEY

I started school at Davenport Elementary School in 1956. The walk to school from my home on Exeter Street took about thirty minutes. I walked past the Soloski and the Anderson homes to Laughton Avenue, and then along to St. Clair Avenue with Gaff's Drug Store at the corner. I felt envy when lunchtime approached, as trays of the small bottles of milk—rich, creamy, homogenized milk! —with the round cardboard lids were brought in for those kids staying at school for lunch.

My walk home was anxiety-filled because of the two older boys who had recently moved onto our street. They were of German descent, which at that time was something to be afraid of as we were just ten years post WWII. They wore thick suede shorts with suspenders and constantly harassed and bullied anyone who came too close to them. We tried to keep our distance but, for whatever reason, they picked on my brother and I. Hans was the older brother, and I can't recall the younger brother's name. They lived five or six houses away on the same side of the street, and the only way to avoid passing their house was to follow a path beside the train tracks that led out to St. Clair Avenue, just north of Caledonia Road; we walked that path many times. Fortunately, Hans and his family moved away at the end of that school year and there was more joy on Exeter Street again.

Other memories return. That damp, cold basement where Brad, my older brother by two years, and I used to box with lightly padded gloves. I remember having at least one bloody nose, but I was never able to hurt him! In the large kitchen that had cracked and broken yellow tiles on the floor, my younger brother Greg pulled a cord from an electric kettle off the stove (he was only about a year old) spilling scalding water onto my foot, which then swelled up like a small yellow balloon. The next day he sat on it and it burst. It wasn't his fault, of course, but I can still feel the stinging pain!

At the top of the stairs leading up to the third floor, there was a small sunroom with wrap-around windows and sheer curtains that only went halfway up, a mottled linoleum floor, some tables with plants on them, a small wooden chair, and one empty square table covered with newspaper and at one end. I remember often seeing my grandpa seated in that chair with a towel around his shoulders and my nana standing behind him with a comb and brush scraping his balding head to get rid of the dandruff. I often sat at the top of the stairs and watched, the sunlight catching the white flakes as they drifted down onto newspaper Nana had spread on the table. Grandpa's eyes would be mostly closed (I had the feeling that he enjoyed this event) but, occasionally, he would open his eyes and glance towards me with a slight smile and a wink, then his eyes would close again. It was amazing how important that wink was to me; it meant he loved me and that I was important to him.

The living room/dining room area was not a large space. It was dark with a thick carpet of dark colours, a long, heavy couch that was also a dark colour, and an old, black dining room table with a white crocheted tablecloth that had three leaves allowing it to expand to seat about ten people. I can only recall one memory of eating at that table with our whole family, and it was an anxiety-provoking experience. We had fish for dinner, which I disliked mainly because of the bones, and I remember noticing my dad starting to cough. He put his hands around his throat, his face turning red and then someone yelled, "He's choking!" I assumed that one of those damn bones from the fish got stuck in his throat. In a split second, my grandfather had a knife in his hand, and he seemed to be putting the knife down my dad's throat as he guided him down to the floor. I was terrified as my nana escorted my brothers and me into the kitchen. The last thing I remember is an ambulance siren, but the anxiety and fear haunted me for a long time. It didn't bode well for my taste for fish either!

My grandfather would take us fishing and, although I liked being in a boat on the water, I hated cramming the poor worms on the hook, taking the hook out of the fish's mouth, and banging it on the head so it would stop flopping around on the bottom of the smelly boat. We were taught how to scrape the scales off, cut the heads off and clean out the insides to prepare for the frying pan.

That memory of when I thought my dad choked on a bone stuck with me for many years, and I had frequent nightmares that he would die from choking on a fish bone. I would remind myself that my dad was okay because I saw him the next day. However, in spite of my mom's empathic abilities, communication in my family regarding emotionally sensitive topics was not one of our strengths! Dad had a rather short fuse. He would get quite angry at what seemed to be normal everyday experiences, such as asking him questions, passing gas in his vicinity, or trying to understand instructions for a game or an item that required assembling

"Oh for God's sake, who wrote these dam instructions anyway?"

So, I was always reluctant to share anything about my "emotional world," knowing that the response would be something along the lines of, "Don't be so silly!" Eventually I did share this dream/memory with my parents, when I was in my late twenties, when Annie and I had them over for dinner one night. When I told them my dream, Mom casually shared that my dad had epilepsy and had a seizure at the table that night! My grandfather put the knife in my dad's mouth to prevent him from biting or swallowing his tongue (that's what they did in the 1950s). I didn't know Dad had epilepsy, but several things began to make sense. I never quite understood why my dad was rarely home when my mom, my brothers and I would have dinner. He would arrive home later, and my mom would sit with him while he ate his dinner. My mom explained that lights, noise, and stress could trigger a seizure, and he wanted to avoid having a seizure in our presence, so he would often have dinner on his own during the week. Looking back, I don't recall my dad ever having another seizure.

One of my favourite memories of Exeter Street is the hot summer afternoons when Brad and I would stand on the street waiting for the large truck that delivered massive blocks of ice to each house for refrigeration. A man would open the back sliding door and give us ice chips that had come off the large ice blocks. They were so cold, so refreshing, on those very hot days. Some important, life-shaping experiences from my time on Exeter Street!

CHAPTER 2

THE MIDDLE YEARS AND ADOLESCENCE

My family moved from the west end of Toronto to 117 Botany Hill Road in Scarborough when I was six, and we lived in a detached, split-level home on a ravine lot. I loved that house and the neighbourhood, particularly the ravine. The long, winding Botany Hill Road followed the top edge of the ravine and ran off Orton Park Road, just north of G. B. Little Public School, coming out again farther north on Orton Park. Orton Park Road was a dead end, and on the west side was a wide-open farmer's field. On the east side of the road there were brand-new homes being constructed, and we played in those buildings for a long time. I can still smell the damp concrete foundations.

Every winter, the community would create a large skating rink in the farmer's field where we would skate and play hockey—when it wasn't too cold! Temperatures back in the late 1950s could dip below -10°F (-23°C) and sometimes down to -25°F (-31°C). There always seemed to be tons of snow to shovel at home and on the skating rink. We would each bring a snow shovel to the rink, line up beside each other across the rink and try to clear that snow (with our skates on!), so we could skate and play hockey. We also enjoyed tobogganing on a winding path in the valley at the end of Orton Park, which was often like a bobsled run. We would frequently see toboggans flying off the path, bodies falling off and tumbling into the snowdrifts to save themselves as toboggans slammed into trees—so exciting! One of the runs was on a winding dirt road that led into the Rouge Valley, and it was nicknamed "Suicide Hill."

In our house, when you walked through our front door, there was a powder room on the left, then a closet and a set of beige carpeted stairs leading up to the three bedrooms and a full bathroom. Straight ahead were two steps down into a large living room with a massive, floor-to-ceiling mirror on the wall to the left. Towards the back of the house, floor-to-ceiling windows looked out onto the ravine. I spent many afternoons sitting at those windows in the orange-coloured swivel rocking chairs. I would watch the squirrels, birds and racoons and play cribbage with my grandpa who had come to live with us after Nana died. He alternated smoking his cigarettes and pipe. When he smoked a cigarette, it would hang down between his lips, the stream of smoke going in and out of his mouth and nose, and every time he would take the cigarette out of his mouth (when counting his cards), there would be a little bit of white paper stuck to his lips, though it didn't seem to bother him! I loved that time with Grandpa.

I spent a great deal of time exploring the ravine that led into the Rouge Valley. The wide variety of trees, bushes, plants, animals, cliffs, creeks, and streams was my place of refuge where I felt "grounded" and "connected" to the world and to the universe. I would walk through the forest, touching leaves, branches and the trunks of trees and wondering how old some of the massive trees were and then thinking about the storms and hurricanes they had endured. When I arrived at the stream we called "Crooked Creek," I would walk along the banks or just sit on a rock and watch the minnows and white suckerfish as they swam in the clear water. I felt a calmness and presence that I am still able to connect with.

One time when I was walking along the bank, I was poking a walking stick I had picked up along the way into the creek bed.

There was a gravelly sound of the stick sinking into the stones and sand at the bottom. As I rounded a bend, I noticed a large brown, furry object floating in the middle of the creek. It was the swollen body of a dog. As it floated by me, I felt so sad. *Do the owners not know where their puppy is?* I wondered. There was nothing I could do, so I continued on my journey, thinking about life and death and wondering if there really was a heaven and hell. I wasn't sure I believed in such places, but I had a powerful sense that it was important to be a good person, to care about others and try to be helpful. I eventually arrived at a large clearing, which was a field of tall hay. The tips brushed across the palms of my hand as I walked the path that led to an empty mansion everyone believed was haunted. I never got closer than about a hundred yards because I was not a big risk taker—why chance it? Without being fully aware of it at the time, I believe this created the foundations of my experience with meditation—sitting, walking, touching, feeling, smelling, and watching the wildlife was my quiet, safe, and healing space!

I was plagued by typical, seasonal allergies (grass, hay, ragweed, animal hair, etc.). Mom put me to bed with cold cloths over my itchy, red, and swollen eyes for hours at a time. She gave me the occasional antihistamine, which would reduce the symptoms enough that I could go to school. I also got many "boils" on various parts of my body that would become quite large, painful, and full of poison. My mother would sit me at the kitchen table, put a generous helping of Rub A535 on a cloth and press it onto the boil (regardless of where it was!). She would hold the cloth in place, gently squeezing applying pressure, determined to extract the poison as quickly as possible. It was like being branded with a hot iron!

"Don't be such a baby!" she would often say, trying to make light of the situation.

Of course, that just made me angry. I sat at that table for hours, crying, squeezing the edge of the table, and feeling the poison being drawn out. A535 was her go-to for almost anything! As painful as it was, it did the job!

The two most impactful experiences from summers spent at Cartwright Point in Kingston where my maternal grandparents lived involve significant fear! When I was about seven, I came upon a rattlesnake and froze. I had witnessed hundreds of snake bites on *Mutual of Omaha's Wild Kingdom* and had been having nightmares about snakes covering my bedroom floor. However, in this situation on the Point, I was fortunate because my grandfather shot it with a .22 rifle. I am still unsure whether this really happened or if it was one of my "lucid dreams," but the nightmares continued. Snakes slithering around my bedroom floor while I laid in my bed every night with the covers pulled tightly over my head. Part of me knew they weren't there, but I couldn't look for a long time. Some nights I actually believed I could hear them slithering!

The second experience was quite traumatic. The family was at a neighbour's BBQ on Cartwright Point, when I was about nine. They had a large yard, like a football field, with a tractor to cut the grass that had the seat attachment separate. The seat attachment had a long steel pole that attached to the actual tractor part. One kid would sit in the seat while three others would lift the steel bar into the air so the one on the seat would tumble backwards, rolling onto the grass and laughing all the way - what great fun! My turn came around, and the anxiety in my stomach rushed through my body—I didn't want to do it! However, between peer pressure and the fear of humiliation and shame if I "wimped out," I got up into the seat. As they hoisted the bar up, I changed my mind and sat forward, and a metal bar smashed into my forehead. I screamed as the blood flowed down my face! I couldn't see, and I just stood there, screaming.

"Oh my God! What happened?" someone yelled.

Within a few seconds, my mom was hysterically yelling my name. I felt her grab me and lift me from the tractor and we fell to the ground. I felt her hand on my forehead and I remember asking her if I was going to die. This, of course, became a humorous story after I returned from the hospital having required only six stiches to close the wound! I have, at times, re-experienced that feeling of peace and contentment that washed over me during the ride to the hospital in my dad's car. Below the tears, I wondered if I was on my way to heaven. Mom was holding me and telling me that everything would be fine, and the words "What will be, will be," came to mind.

When I was eleven, I used to play war in the ravine with two close friends, Chris and Peter. After a few skirmishes and we emerged victorious, we would holster our stick guns and go to someone's house for a snack. One day, Peter and I had gotten into an argument, and I called him names and pushed him to the ground. He ran home crying. I felt bad about that, but it was his fault!

The next day, Peter's mom knocked on our front door and my mom answered. I lurked in the living room to hear what was being said. After a few minutes, my mom came into the living room and asked me what had happened with Peter the day before. I explained the argument, including the name-calling and pushing him down. My mom was not happy and told me that I had to go to Peter's house and apologize. As a fairly obedient child, I reluctantly marched around the corner, feeling that anxiety welling up from the pit of my stomach. My heart pounding, I knocked on their side door, and Peter's mom answered but did not invite me in. I wanted to get this over with as soon as possible so I simply said, "I'm sorry for hurting Peter." With tears in her eyes, an angry expression on her face and her voice quivering, she said, "Peter is my only son, and it upsets me to see him hurt. Please don't do that again." With tears in my eyes, I said, "I'm sorry and I promise I won't do that again.".

On the walk home, two things were clear to me: that I would do my best not to treat anyone like that again, and that I did not want to play with Peter anymore! However, I realized how important friendships are and that friends will come and go. I became interested in peer relationships and often found myself on the periphery of different groups of friends, observing the ways they interacted with each other. I recall watching as the bullies in class would tease and ridicule a boy named Jan who lived with cerebral palsy. They would also make fun of the one Jewish boy in the class and the two brothers who were of First Nations descent (Ojibwa), who later became two of my best friends.

The notion of death and the experience of loss became a focus for me. I was twelve years old when my nana died. Mom woke up my brothers and me one morning and said that Nana had died that night, so they had to go to be with Grandpa and "Take care of things." The fact that my brothers and I did not go was how my parents tried to protect us from the pain of losing someone so dear to us. Unfortunately, that just made it harder to share painful emotions because we understood the message to be, "Sort out those emotions yourself and move on."

I was angry on my way to school that morning and then broke down in tears during first period. Mrs. Lawrence, probably my favourite elementary school teacher, was a warm, affectionate woman, and she hugged me and walked me to the office, where I stayed for the remainder of the period. The principal asked if I wanted to go home, but I knew my parents were not there. I knew I needed to be stronger as I did not want them to contact my parents. I thought about how sad my dad was to lose his mom, and I stopped crying and returned to class. All heads turned in my direction. I assumed that Mrs. Lawrence had told the class that my grandmother died, and it felt very awkward. No one said anything, not even the bullies in class. Death had a silencing effect on them too!

I was at home sick and watching TV that November when the news came on that President John F. Kennedy had been shot. There were scenes of scores of people outside the hospital where he had been taken and it looked like everyone was crying. I instinctively started to cry because of a deep sense of loss and fear I felt in the pit of my stomach. Something very bad had happened and we would never be the same. It was so very sad, particularly when they showed the motorcade, the shot he took to the head and Jackie climbing onto the trunk to retrieve something. I'd held JFK in high regard; his voice resonated within me then, and to this day I can still hear that Boston accent.

On one very hot summer evening when I was fourteen, my friends and I were sitting on the front porch on Botany Hill when we heard an ambulance approaching. As it sped by us and rounded the corner heading west towards Orton Park Road, the siren became silent. We could still see the flashing lights, so we knew it had stopped at someone's house around the corner. We all walked hurriedly around the bend to see the attendants bring a stretcher out of a house with a body on it that was covered completely—not a good sign! We later found out that a boy who went to our school had died from propane poisoning. The story that got shared throughout the school was that he had a dentist appointment the next day, was terrified of the dentist and decided to knock himself out with propane so he didn't have to go to the appointment.

The adults didn't suspect he had tried to kill himself, as there was no note and he had not appeared depressed to anyone in his family or anyone at school. However, my memory of him was that he was a loner, a science enthusiast, and he was routinely bullied. My closest friends and I thought it was more likely he just didn't want to be alive anymore, but this was 1965 and no one openly talked about such things! I had several disturbing dreams for a few weeks following his death. Some dreams involved seeing him with the propane tank, often crying and breathing in the gas, and other dreams were about his mom and dad being alone in the home just sitting at the kitchen table, not talking—just in shock at the loss of their only son. When I woke from such dreams, I was thankful to be alive.

My maternal grandfather died at age sixty-four when his car went off a bridge in Kingston, Ontario; he had a heart attack. I was sixteen and quite close with him. He had a great sense of humour and, when we were younger, tickled us until we cried. He shifted to teasing us when we were older—all in good fun! My maternal grandmother was a sweet but strange woman during those years. She did not talk a lot, and she had some interesting rituals when she would cook, clean, iron clothing or knit. I remember watching her intentionally because she made odd gestures with her hands and arms from time to time. At first, I thought she was shooing flies away until I realized there were no flies! Her hands and arms would make circling gestures in front of her and around her head. I never quite understood what that was about, and I was not going to ask! I found out later that she had experienced what was termed a "nervous breakdown," was hospitalized and I learned years later that she received electric shock treatments which apparently helped lift a significant, long-standing depression.

Despite the tractor incident from earlier, we were fortunate to be able to spend vacation time with my maternal grandparents at their home on Cartwright Point, which was right on the St. Lawrence River. There were several neighbours with children around our age, so we had friends and a number of homes we could visit. We swam in the river every day. There was a wooden dock that had an old metal rowboat with oars that had seen better days. There was also an old shiny wooden inboard motorboat, and you could always smell the gas mixed with the smell of a few dead sunfish!

When I stood on the sandy beach looking across the river towards New York, I saw the homes of Cartwright Point to my left and massive rocks one hundred yards to my right where the waves would wash in and crash violently against the rocks. We used to walk along the beach and then climb the rocks about a mile out to a peninsula, from here we could see Old Fort Henry. I can still hear the cannons that fired every day at five pm. So, my grandfather's death brought back all kinds of memories—awake and in my dreams.

Following the path that led to the beach from my grandparent's home down the hill and across the dirt road, I can still feel the heat from the summer sun and smell the tall wheatgrass that rose above my head. The waves crashed into the rocks on windy days and rolled up onto the sand on calm days. I still recall the smell of wax mixed with gas from the mahogany inboard motorboat and the faint smell of dead sunfish that often washed up on shore. Standing on the wooden dock and listening to the sounds from the waves, the seagulls flying overhead and the faint horns from the cargo ships that travelled the St. Lawrence, I always felt a relaxed calm move through me. It is another of my "quiet spaces" I can drop into anytime and anywhere by simply following my breath!

I have vivid memories of visiting my Aunt and Uncle's cottage on Georgian Bay. It was a lovely cottage, and I sometimes enjoyed hanging out with my cousins who were of similar age, but I often felt nauseous because of the constant smell of my uncle's ubiquitous cigars. All the other adults smoked cigarettes as well. We were all in the water at the end of their dock one day while my uncle was getting the boat ready for skiing. I was on one side of the dock in the waist-deep water, and my older brother and cousins were on the other side. Out of the corner of my eye, I saw something move. When I turned to look, there was a long, mottled snake coming towards me! Anyone who has ever tried to run in waist-deep water knows how slow one moves, but I took three giant leaps and I was on the shore.

"Don't worry, it's only a water moccasin—it won't hurt you," my uncle yelled.

I never went back in that water again! My snake phobia remained a nightly struggle and became increasingly powerful. The thoughts of snakes would come into my awareness as I brushed my teeth before bed and pictured a few slithering under my bed. When I finished brushing my teeth, I would feel those butterflies in my stomach. My breathing became increasingly rapid and then I would run to my room, leap into bed, pull the covers over my head and begin to quiver. More and more snakes slithered on the floor under my bed. This went on nightly until I was about twelve but weakened as my rational mind became increasingly stronger. I always keep a close eye on rocks and bushes when I walk in nature to this day; you never know when a snake might appear!

Other vivid memories were around the "drives"! My dad loved fast convertibles. The two I remember were both Chevy Impala convertibles with the most powerful engines. The last one was a 1967 gold Impala that had a 396-turbojet engine—I burned a lot of rubber off those tires! Both my parents were smokers, and I can still see my mom in the front passenger seat placing two cigarettes in her mouth, lighting them (in the wind!) and passing one to my dad as he drove. I can smell the smoke, which I found comforting at the time. Dad loved to drive fast, tailgate and pass as many vehicles as he could. The most recurring feeling when I recall those drives is fear! I watched closely as he would get closer and closer to a car ahead, and I could feel my feet press down on the floor of the car as if I could slow the car down! I could see Mom's legs tighten as she pushed back on the seat. My heart pounding I would pray silently, "Please God, let us get there alive!"

Elementary school was primarily a social event for me, and I was never worried or concerned about grades. I did the work required in class, but my focus was always watching the other kids and how they interacted. I was primarily on the sidelines, shy and introverted, watching the stories play out between classmates and teachers. I had developed a connection with that part of me that could step outside of my immediate experience and look at what was happening in the various sub stories of my life. I recall a few teachers who truly seemed to care, but many more who were self-important, power-hungry bullies who controlled their classes through intimidation and fear, shame, and humiliation. There would often be at least one student writing lines on the chalkboard that said "I must not swear in class" or the like. At least one student would be standing at their desk, arms outstretched and one hand, palm up, holding a book (a standard punishment at the time). There was always at least one student standing with their face buried in a corner of the class. I had my turns at each of these areas and on two occasions was sent to the principal's office to get "the strap"—like the long, brown leather straps that Barber's used to sharpen their razors. That was the strap that Mr. Lehman (my French teacher in Grade 6) used because I did what he told me to do! That's right, I did what he asked and got three strikes on the palm of each of my hands for it. He had asked me a question that I did not hear, and he yelled, "Hunter, wave your arms, stomp your feet—do something to show you're alive!" So, I waved my arms and stomped my feet. Classmates laughed, but not the teacher! He leapt over an empty desk, smacked my head, grabbed my sweater at the back of my neck and "escorted" me to the office, where I received the strap. Not a nice man!

I had a bit of a temper in my younger years, but it took a lot of provocation for me to "snap" I once attacked a boy at school who had been teasing me constantly for weeks on end. One day he was walking backwards about six feet in front of me and telling me how stupid I was, so I charged him, wrapped my hands around his throat and pushed him to the ground. I was clearly stronger than him, and I thought, *this is stupid!* So, I got off him and told him to leave me alone; he never spoke to me again.

Another time, my friends and I were deep in the ravine with all our "weapons"—pellet rifles, bean guns and knives—all of which were primarily for target practice. One of my friends decided to start shooting the "beans," which sting when they hit skin at me. I repeatedly told him to stop, and when he didn't, I snapped, pulled my six-inch Bowie knife from its sheath and threw it at him, aiming just in front of his feet, where it landed. He was not impressed, shouted a few choice words at me and left. He eventually got over it, and he never pushed me like that again.

The intensity of my anger scared me as well, and I knew I had to develop better controls. No more knives and guns for me!

I always managed to pass each school year without doing much work outside of the classrooms—or even in them! There was a consistent pattern between grades two and six. After first term my grades ranged between 35 and 60 percent, with English and math consistently on the higher end simply because I enjoyed them. The first term would come to an end with parent/teacher interviews, during which time my parents would hear that I clowned around far too much, didn't pay attention in class and rarely completed my homework. If I didn't "smarten up," I would not pass my year. My parents were always understandably disappointed after these meetings and would tell me to try harder, but they never pressured me. I would pull my socks up and earn grades between 50 and 60 in the second term, which pleased my parents and got teachers off my back. I continued in this fashion through to the end of each year and happily went on to the next grade.

I never found the work hard and didn't read an entire book until the last term of Grade 8, when we were going to have a test in English worth 50 percent on a novel. *Black Like Me* by John Howard Griffin is about a white man from Texas who had his skin temporarily darkened and travelled through the southern United States to experience the effects of racism and segregation firsthand. This was a turning point, and I began to enjoy reading and became obsessed with racism. I read anything I could find, especially material written by African Americans, such as "Soul on Ice" by Eldridge Cleaver (1968) and "Black Power" by Stokely Carmichael and Charles Hamilton (1967). I was finding an outlet for my anger, those who oppress others! Communist governments in North Vietnam, Russia, China, the many Dictatorships around the world, and our own treatment of Native Indians, became the focus of my anger and rage.

Chronic Pain: My Journey

In a parent/teacher interview during second term in Grade 8, the principal informed my parents that I could never complete an academic stream in high school, and I should consider a four-year technical program. My parents supported the plan, even though most of my friends were going to a different high school in the academic stream.

Cedarbrae Collegiate in Scarborough was well-known for its technical programs, and because of the recommendations from my former principal, I was enrolled in the four-year program. This turned out to be four years of frustration, anger and resentment. There were so many racist bullies, students and some teachers, whose primary strategy for holding onto power and control was through emotional abuse and humiliation.

Socially, I remained connected to my previous peer groups. I had developed relationships with two different groups of friends. One group of boys was socially appropriate, kind, considerate and respectful of the adult world, the other enjoyed getting drunk, gambling and chasing after girls. After being teased and bullied by some of this latter group from grades six to eight, part of me felt privileged to be accepted, but I never felt like I belonged. I was always anxious and on edge around them, but they could be very persuasive when they wanted me to take part in their "antics."

When we were sixteen, we met almost every Friday and Saturday evening following our shift at the Busy Bee grocery store in Orton Park Plaza. We would go to one of two houses where parents were not often home, drink a lot of alcohol, smoke cigarettes and play poker for money. I usually lost. These friends were also "speed demons" in their parents' cars, and I constantly prepared myself for death; seat belts were not mandatory at that time. They were always speeding, smoking, and hanging out the windows yelling at girls walking down the street, which made me feel uncomfortable and embarrassed.

One night we went to the drive-in to see *Bullet* with Steve McQueen, which included many scenes of stunt driving. One friend drove his father's Dodge Charger, and on the way home from the movie, he believed he was Steve McQueen. We reached 130 mph on the highway. He pulled off onto a small county road that was deserted and did multiple donuts while I grasped the back of the passenger seat, my heart beating out of my chest as the adrenaline flowed through my body. I was terrified! That memory is so strong that I still connect to that nausea in the pit of my stomach to this day.

I had several other terrifying experiences in my friend Gerry's red Mustang that belonged to his father. He got a kick out of taunting the police! We were careening west on Ellesmere Road one evening travelling around 80 mph when we flew past an officer standing beside his cruiser with a speed gun. Within seconds, the officer was in his cruiser and a chase began. I thought I was going to have a heart attack! Gerry flew around corners and through the side streets, tires squealing, and eventually pulled into a parking lot full of cars. He parked the car and waited for twenty minutes, and when there was no sign of the police, we drove home. When he dropped me off, he was giggling.

"See you tomorrow," he said as I exited the car.

"You are fucking crazy man!" I yelled at him.

"I know!" he yelled as he sped away, tires squealing.

My other friends were much easier to be around. They were primarily into music, sports, smoking marijuana, experimenting with mescaline, LSD and mushrooms. They were fully engaging in the hippie movement—love, peace and rock 'n' roll! I was happier and more relaxed with this group, and I still don't understand why I continued to hang out with the other group. Likely the risk-taking. As mentioned before, we hunted (with pellet guns) every weekend, primarily mice, squirrels, and some birds (I still feel sick when I think about this now!).

My relationship with the more dangerous group came to an end one weekend in the summer of 1966. Our part-time jobs at The Busy Bee meant we had money for poker, cigarettes, alcohol, and gas for those who had their own cars. They decided we were going to Buffalo to see the stock car races, and their shopping list included four cases of beer and half a dozen bottles of liquor! I immediately knew this was a terrible idea and did not want to go, but, as I said, they could be persuasive. I decided that if I was going to go, I wanted someone with me that I trusted, so I asked Jim, from my other group, to come along. It took some convincing because he disliked most of the boys, but he agreed.

There were two cars with four guys in each car, and the alcohol was equally divided between the two cars. Most of it was in the trunks and wrapped in blankets and sleeping bags, except for one case of beer that was to be consumed during the drive to Buffalo (yes, across the border!). The speed limit on the highways in 1966 was 100 mph, and we routinely exceeded 120 mph. Oh, and there was no designated driver! Jim and I were in the back seat of Gerry's Mustang struggling with anxiety and panic as Gerry and his buddy in the front continued to guzzle beer as we drove!

When we arrived in Buffalo, Jim and I thought we were heading to the racetrack, but our hearts sank when we pulled into the parking lot of a local bar. Jim and I both noted the rather large young men wearing "army" T-shirts, and we decided to stay in the mustang while the others went into the bar for a beer. Ten minutes later, our friends came running out of the bar with at least ten large angry men in chase. This eventful night ended in a car chase through the streets of Buffalo! Gerry took one turn after another trying to evade our pursuers. Our other friends were in Doug's Dodge Charger, and we lost them within minutes. I had never seen Gerry scared, but he was terrified at that point. In retrospect, it seems we all thought we were going to die that night. We were saved by a train that was approaching from our right; we could see the tracks ahead. Gerry put the gas pedal to the floor and flew over the tracks just as the guard rails were lowering. Our pursuers were blocked. As he had done before, Gerry sped through a number of side streets and pulled in behind a small convenience store, where we sat in silence for what seemed like an hour. Then Gerry opened another beer.

"Okay boys, let's go home."

Although he drank a couple of beers on that drive home, he did stay within the speed limit!

From that point on, I only hung out with my core group of friends, Mike, Bev, Wayne, Ian, Chris, John and Jim. We truly enjoyed each other's company, spending many hours in Mike's basement smoking marijuana, playing table hockey, and engaging in deep, philosophical, existential conversations. That is, Wayne and I engaged in such conversations while sitting on the large sofa while the others played table hockey with abandon! Under the influence of the marijuana, they became hockey players, while Wayne and I sunk back into the soft dark brown couch and just talked.

"Oh man, can you believe those Americans, fighting that stupid fucking war in Vietnam?" I said, as I took another drag on a joint and passed it to Wayne.

"Ya well, the war is one big fuck-up, but what about how black people and Indians are treated in their own country—that's a bigger problem." Wayne took a drag from the joint, and passing it on said, "Glad we live here man."

We were very connected with the whole peace, love and rock 'n' roll right down to the torn jeans, love beads and bare feet. In the summer of 1966 I remember walking everywhere in bare feet, carrying our guitars, heading to the ravine to "jam." We would run connecting extension cords from a friend's house at the top of a hill, down to a makeshift stage where drums and amplifiers were arranged. Very fond memories, as music became increasingly important in my life – I was able to connect with my "quiet space" again.

As high school wore on, it became clear that I had few technical skills. I was taking shop subjects—auto mechanics, woodworking, electricity, etc.—and scoring between 40 and 55 percent. I even had two teachers who said that if I agreed to never take that class again, they would give me a pass! I'd almost severed the teacher's hand on the lathe in woodworking and come close to electrocuting our electricity teacher, so that was probably for the best. However, in my academic subjects I was consistently achieving grades between 70 and 85 percent, and I was enjoying some of those classes.

During eleventh grade, I was having an increasingly difficult time getting along with classmates (many of whom were incredibly racist and sexist) and most of my teachers. I was not enjoying school at all, but I reminded myself that I only had one more year. During the summer of 1967, much of our world was focused on the inhumane treatment of people of colour (including American and Canadian Indians) and the Vietnam war. It's safe to say that we were angry about injustice, war, and our patriarchal society, and we blamed it on our parents' generation. I returned to Grade 12 that September in a very negative frame of mind, and I was unhappy with the subjects and teachers I had for that first semester. At the end of that September, I had an argument with my English teacher, a bully who believed he was right about everything. He became frustrated when I argued that everyone is entitled to have their own opinion and that his opinion was not always right.

"How could you get to Grade 12 and still be so damned stupid, Hunter?" he asked.

I was sensitive to people thinking I was stupid, so I dropped my books on the floor and replied, "How could you get to your age and be such an asshole?" Then I walked out of his class and out of the school, never to return!

I was terrified of telling my parents that I quit school, particularly my dad.

"Oh, you stupid ass!" my mom said, which I expected.

My dad, however, surprised me when he said, "So, what's your plan now?"

We talked about working and perhaps travelling. He was able to get my job back in the shipping room at Gestetner (paper goods, printing supplies, duplicating machines, etc.), where I worked for over a year, saving some money to travel. I fantasized about travelling through the British Isles and Europe as I carried out my shipping duties day after day. I quickly realized that I did not want to work in a shipping room my whole life, and I began contemplating returning to school.

CHAPTER 3

WHAT TO DO

My older brother Brad was attending Centennial College and was heavily into philosophy and Buddhism, meditating routinely. He frequently offered counsel and support as I struggled with what to do with my life. I recall several conversations with him about the racial oppression experience in America and the Buddhist perspectives on the meaning of life and death. He taught me how to meditate and turned me onto important literature at the time—Martin Luther King, Eldridge Cleaver, Malcolm X, and the Black Panthers. I proudly displayed posters of them on the walls in my bedroom, along with Jimi Hendrix and Janice Joplin!

Through Brad's help with the art of meditation, I eventually realized the importance of my own quiet, calm space inside, and I spent time there daily as I walked through the ravine. I was experiencing what Thomas Moore referred to as my true "original self." *The Three Pillars of Zen* by Philip Kapleau became my Bible for many years. I felt strong, balanced, and connected to the world at large, and philosophy, spirituality and psychology became my obsession. I frequently sat by large trees that lined the bank of the creek, meditating with the sounds of the water flowing, the breeze blowing and the sounds of animals communicating. Another favourite spot for meditation was an open field close to train tracks. During these experiences, I began to realize the power of my mind. I experienced significant changes in bodily sensations and even felt like time slowed down. I truly felt "at one" with the universe!

I also met a lovely young lady, Linda, who was the first girl I ever dated. I became totally focused on her and our developing relationship, as I felt shocked that a girl was interested in me romantically. But something felt a little off. I knew in my heart that she was not the one I wanted to spend my life with. I was not at all clear about the kind of girl I was looking for, as I had precious little experience with girls.

After a year of saving, I decided it was time to travel, and I connected with Gerry the speed demon again. He was also interested in travelling and worked at Gestetner as well; he had mellowed a little by that time. We decided we wanted to see England, Scotland and France. There was a deep part of me that was particularly anxious about this trip because of a little separation anxiety mixed with Gerry's history of risk-taking, but I had made the plans and felt I had to follow through.

This turned out to be both bad timing and the wrong person to travel with. As our 747 out of Pearson Airport flew over Montreal, there was significant turbulence, and the plane began to turn sharply. The pilot informed us there was a problem with one of the engines and said we had to return to Toronto after dumping most of our fuel in Lake Ontario because we couldn't land with a full tank. As we circled the lake, I could hear and feel the fuel being released. Once we landed and transferred to another plane, I still hadn't shaken that knowing feeling inside that this was a bad idea, but I pushed on.

I had decided to part ways with Gerry, as I had a specific destination in Scotland (friends of the family in Glasgow), and he was intent on heading to Europe. From London, I took the train to Scotland and met up with the family friends, with whom I stayed for a fortnight. I was not in a good space—anxiety was having its way with me! I was questioning decisions I had made regarding work and school and was unsure of where my life was going. The balance and strength I had seemed to disappear.

However, there was a part of me that felt like I was home. I experienced a similar feeling in Grade 7 when our history teacher put on a film of the Battle of Culloden in 1746. I had this eerie, déjà vu feeling that I had been there. I loved the countryside in Scotland and was blessed to have friends in Glasgow who took me in, fed me and tried desperately to entertain me. One of my hosts announced that they were to be off to Aberdeen for the World Pipe Band Championships and invited me to go along. That was such an incredible experience, as I was able to ride with the pipe band in their bus, listening to them practice and fool around. I had a real struggle hearing what they said because of their thick accents (and likely my hearing!). When we returned from Aberdeen, I became homesick and decided to return home without going to France. I was back home in three weeks, which was supposed to be three months!

Prior to this trip, I had met Annie, the youngest daughter of my parents' closest friends, Don and Marg. It was New Year's Eve and my parents traditionally played bridge with Don and Marg. I had been out with friends and returned home just after midnight. As I entered the house, I heard voices singing "Big Yellow Taxi," and there was Annie and her friend Bonnie sitting on the living room floor playing guitars and singing. My mom and dad were clearly feeling the Myers's Rum and were singing along. As I entered and caught sight of Annie, something in her eyes touched me deeply. I couldn't look away, and I was convinced I needed to see her again!

I struggled, during my meditations with what I realized were some important decisions. I had many conversations with my best friend at the time, Wayne, who always supported whatever I decided. After taking an achievement test (CAT) to determine if I would have to take any courses to upgrade (I didn't), I returned as an advanced student to the three-year Child and Youth Care Program at Centennial College in Scarborough.

I also decided that Annie was the person I wanted to spend more time with, so I ended my relationship with Linda. Annie was attending the York Regional Nursing School that was connected to North York General Hospital. I was driving a delivery truck for Gestetner, and the nursing school was one of my stops. On one of my deliveries, I saw her and we chatted briefly. I had always been painfully shy and had few social skills, but Annie was the opposite. Perhaps that was one of the many things I found attractive about her. As I was still working in the dead-end shipping room at Gestetner, my self-esteem was at a low point, I was worried about how college would play out. I was fortunate to run into her again at the nursing school while making a delivery and we finally began dating. I was a tiny bit obsessive about calling her every evening at 7:00 p.m., a phone call which I later found out she routinely dreaded. I was not much of a conversationalist, but I was determined and persevered!

An increasing number of young people in our Scarborough community were becoming involved in street gangs. Wayne and I decided we could help by opening a space for young people in our area to go in the evenings instead of hanging around in small plazas, malls and schoolyards. We had heard about a youth group being held at St. Mark's, the local United Church, so we decided to check it out one evening. There were a handful of youth between the ages of twelve and seventeen spread out across the basement floor that looked like a gym with a stage at the end. A young man announced they were electing a new president and vice president of the group, so Wayne and I nominated each other, gave a brief impromptu speech about what we could do in this space and were voted into office. We convinced other friends to participate as well, which gave us about thirty-five young people in the group.

Wayne and I met with our closest friends Chris, Mike and Ian to brainstorm ideas about how we would draw other young people in. We were into music—playing, singing, and writing (my wished-for extroverted side!)—so we decided to write and mount a musical production. This was a life-changing experience for me. We announced this plan to the wider youth group, and we held auditions and cast the play, which was set in medieval times. We imagined the set for our play to be in the nave upstairs, so we approached the church elders for permission. Surprisingly, they agreed.

Annie and I became close with our friends Barb and Elton (RIP), and I very much enjoyed reading stories to their eldest daughter Vanessa during that time. Elton was the smartest person I ever knew, and his memory and retention ability were truly second to none. He was over six feet tall, lanky, with a beard and mustache; he was a handsome man. Elton directed our play, and he became my best friend. One of my philosophy professors from college, Fred Booker, was a gifted singer and worked with me intensely when the lead backed out and I was thrown into the fire to replace him. I had three solos, and it was only because of Fred that I was able to stay on key. Thank you, Fred!

We received positive responses from the audience who filled the church. I wish we had arranged to do at least two shows, but we only performed that one evening. I was eighteen, and that night I felt my parents were proud of me. As I stood on the platform bowing with the whole cast, the crowd of about one hundred stood, applauding. Tears streamed down my face—I had never felt anything like that before. After the cast bowed, I invited Elton to stand up as our director, which he did—reluctantly! As the applause faded and people were coming up to congratulate us, John McDonaugh (another philosophy professor from Centennial College) gave me a hug before he headed for the door. My mom was approaching, also tearful, and John stopped her and said, "Let him enjoy this. It's a once in a lifetime experience." My mom's expression of pride and joy in that moment has stayed with me; it felt so good to have my parents show how proud they were. The only other time I recall them showing pride in something I accomplished was when I swam competitively in my early adolescence. I appreciate those moments!

College was truly inspiring. I had some amazing professors in philosophy (John, Betty-Ann, Thomas and Fred), sociology (Bob) and psychology (Abe), and, without too much effort, I did very well. Working with young people and families who were struggling was exactly what I wanted to do, and I was totally invested in reading and learning as much as I possibly could about the field of counselling and psychotherapy. Joel and Brian were our two primary teachers in Child and Youth Work, and I enjoyed all the courses immensely. But it was my placements at Whitby Psychiatric Hospital with adolescents and Scarborough General Hospital's 3040 Clinic that cemented my love for the field.

The adolescent unit was my first field placement in my second year at Centennial College in the Child and Youth Worker program. On my first day of placement, I was confronted with an angry, out of control sixteen-year-old girl who was heading for the front door as staff were yelling, "Stop her!" She was coming right at me, and I suspected she would run right over me. I dropped my coffee cup on the floor, spun around, latched onto her shoulders, and pulled her down onto the floor into the restraint hold we had been taught. I sat with my back against a wall, her seated between my legs, her back to me. My hands held her wrists and I crossed her arms across her chest, my chin tucked into the crook of her neck. I held on tightly as she continued to scream and struggle to get loose. I recall thinking, *Calm, soft, gentle but firm*, so I gently repeated phrases that would let her know that it was okay, that I was with her, that she was safe, and that it was okay to calm down and get back in control.

Thirty minutes later, I felt her body starting to relax, and she stopped screaming. I could still feel the rage in her and I thought that if I let her go now, she would bolt, so I held on for another fifteen minutes, softly explaining that she needed to let me know she had regained control and would not run when I let go. I had never been so exhausted! Her assigned staff were close by and praised her for regaining control, saying they would take her back to her room when she was ready. My inclination was to stay with this patient as she regained control and have a proper "debriefing," which was the protocol we learned, but it also felt very much like an imperative! Her staff agreed to allow me to debrief with her along with her primary staff. I was able to develop a positive, therapeutic relationship with this young person and most of the other youth I worked with in that program. I learned then that these young people knew when their staff were being genuine!

My relationship with Annie grew stronger over my three years of college, and we began talking about marriage. I asked her to marry me numerous times, but she would just chuckle and say we should wait until after college. So, in 1973, with both of us scheduled to graduate the following year, she finally said "yes." I had secured a position with the adolescent unit at Whitby Psychiatric Hospital, and Annie got a nursing position on a medical unit at Centenary Hospital (now Rouge Valley) in Scarborough. The years from 1969 through to 1981 (from the age of eighteen to thirty) were the happiest years of my life.

CHAPTER 4

CAREER AND FAMILY

I consistently made a point of connecting with the most experienced professionals in my field but also in social work and particularly psychiatry. I wanted to become the most knowledgeable and effective therapist I could be. At Whitby Psychiatric Hospital, I learned a great deal about individual and group psychotherapy from Dr. Jim Ricks, and a great deal about families from Alan Vallillee, a truly gifted social worker. This early learning experience allowed me to develop a clinical foundation for my counselling skills.

These experiences laid the foundation for my understanding of transference and countertransference, as I struggled to understand my own reactions to the youth and families I worked with, as well as to my colleagues. At twenty, I was only a few years older that many of the youth admitted to the adolescent unit. I had reactions, positive and negative, and I was determined to understand the ways in which they impacted my therapeutic work. I learned how some interventions led to positive therapeutic relationships, while others created impossible divides. It was a painful learning experience to watch staff relate to the young patients in ways that too often triggered negative responses. There was a powerful lingering attitude amongst some staff that these youth had anger and rage they needed to get out and it was their job to help them release it. Some staff appeared to intentionally antagonize patients to get them to "blow"—to become furious and act out to the extent that they had to be physically restrained and most often medicated with 25 mg of chlorpromazine (IM). The Adolescent Cottage at Whitby was two stories, had ten bedrooms, two bathrooms, a "quiet room" (isolation room), a nursing station, and a full kitchen, dining room and TV room. We often had six to eight girls and six to eight boys living in this space. The main floor had a large games room, living room and offices.

I realized that just listening to patients' stories, validating their experiences, and offering hope were the three most important aspects of developing a therapeutic alliance. It also became painfully clear that the attitudes and reactions from staff frequently triggered hostility and rage in these young people making any therapeutic alliance with them impossible. During the two years I was involved in that program, most of our patients had been through multiple treatment settings and obtained multiple diagnoses including psychoses, oppositional defiant disorders, conduct disorders, etc. Many of the youth were "Crown Wards of the Children's Aid Society after being apprehended from their families, because of abuse and neglect. The patients who did have families were often part of chaotic, conflict-ridden systems that required long-term interventions. This became increasingly discouraging for me, as there appeared to be little hope that they would receive the ongoing help they required to improve their relationships and survive as a family unit.

I was offered a permanent night position at Whitby, which I gratefully accepted, as I had moved out of my parent's home and needed the income. In my third and final year of the CYW program, I went to the director and asked if my time working at Whitby could be accepted as my final placement.

"You want your cake and to eat it as well, but that's not going to happen" he said. "Besides, nights is not an active shift."

"Nights is often the most active shift," I said in disbelief.

However, I still had to complete a final placement, which I secured at Scarborough General Hospital's 3040 Clinic. Every

Monday, Tuesday and Wednesday, I worked at Whitby from 11:30 p.m. to 7:30 a.m, raced to be at the 3040 Clinic by 8:30 a.m., worked until 5:00 p.m., and then tried to sleep for a couple of hours before having to drive back to Whitby for my night shift. This went on for six months until I graduated in June of 1974.

After graduation, I stayed at Whitby Psychiatric Hospital for another year, and what a year it was! I continued to work nights, which were quite active. I learned so much about the impact of "contagion" and explored a variety of techniques for preventing all-out war in the cottage. One or more patients would escalate a few times a week, and with their adrenaline pumping and their anger growing, physically moving them to the "quiet room" (isolation) was key to preventing contagion from setting in. Easier said than done, as there was only two child and youth counsellors (usually a male and a female) in the cottage and a hospital nursing supervisor on call.

One nightmare incident happened at change of shift (around 11:45 p.m.). My co-worker and I were heading upstairs while the evening staff prepared to leave. We could hear crying and yelling from the bedroom area—evening staff were supposed to ensure the patients were settled for the night—and when we got to the nursing station, we heard a window smash. One patient had broken her window and cut her wrist with a piece of the glass. We pulled her into the nursing station and began to bandage her wrist and try to calm her down when we heard another window break. I ran down the hall and found a second patient who had smashed her window and had cut her forearm, which was bleeding profusely. I did not want to take her to the nursing station where the other patient was, so I took her downstairs to the main office. I was happy to see that two of the evening staff had not left yet, and I asked one of them to care for this patient's wound and the other to return upstairs to keep all the other patients settled. Everyone was awake now! I went from room to room, providing reassurance that we had everything under control, and everyone was okay. I had managed to develop a positive relationship with the oldest youth, who were helpful in establishing calm.

We had to page the nursing supervisor two to four times a week to have them come to the cottage with a "shot" (25 mg of chlorpromazine) to help a young out-of-control patient settle. Some supervisors had more compassion than others. One night when we held a fourteen-year-old girl face down on the floor of the quiet room to stop her from running into the walls, the nursing supervisor (a male) casually walked into the room, stood over the fully clothed patient and said, "Oh darling, causing trouble again I see?" He then launched the syringe from a standing position, piercing the patient's jeans on her buttocks. The nurse depressed the syringe, withdrew it and slapped the patient's buttocks saying, "There you go, darling. That should settle you down."

"Why would you throw the needle and smack the patient's butt?" I asked in utter shock.

"It gets the medication flowing quicker," he said as he left the quiet room.

That night helped me decide I could not work in this environment much longer, and I was fortunate to land a much sought-after position with the Child and Family Studies Centre at the Clarke Institute of Psychiatry (now CAMH) in Toronto. As I had done at Whitby, I made it my mission to connect with the best psychiatrists, psychologists, and social workers I could find and learn as much as I possibly could from them about assessment, case formulation and treatment. I approached each of them independently and requested direct clinical supervision, which they were all quite happy to provide. Drs Leon Sloman, Sam Izenberg, Susan Bradley, Chris Webster, Mary Konstantareas and Jeremy Harmon were my dream team of mentors! I became a part of several multidisciplinary teams engaged in individual, group and family therapy with all ages of children and youth living with a broad range of disorders. In addition to my clinical experience,

I participated in research, publication, and presentations of our work. I was definitely in my element.

During my tenure at the Clarke, I became aware of a significant problem with my hearing. We worked in teams and, while one or two members carried out a family assessment, the rest of us (usually three or four other team members) watched and listened from behind the one-way mirror. I realized I needed to see people's lips moving and facial expressions to know what they were saying. I had no idea what people with their backs to me were saying as my hearing was significantly impaired. Following an audiology assessment, I was told that I had significant hearing loss in both ears in the higher frequencies and I was likely experiencing tinnitus (ringing in the ears), particularly at night. The hearing loss meant I had a trouble identifying consonants, which carry the meaning in words, so words that rhymed were a real problem!

I became skilled at lipreading and analyzing facial expressions and other non-verbal communication. I came to understand several experiences from my youth that made me wonder if I always had this hearing loss. Teachers and family members consistently hounded me about "not listening," which often got me into trouble. I could not make out most of the lyrics in songs on the radio, even though I loved music, singing and playing guitar. Mom told me repeatedly, "You must be tone deaf, you really can't stay on key." My confidence shaken; I became reluctant to sing in front of others. When I would read the actual lyrics in print, I was constantly blown away — "I had no idea that's what the song was about!"

To add to possible causal factors of hearing loss and tinnitus, my dad had a habit of "cuffing us in the ear," as he phrased it. If we did anything that triggered his annoyance (giving attitude, burping, or farting) and we were within reach, he would slap us on the side of the head, across the ear. Although this didn't hurt much, I remember my ears ringing for days after a swat! To be fair to my dad, this practice stopped once we hit adolescence and our relationship became much more positive. But, frequent ear, nose and throat infections, along with the frequent ringing in the ears likely had a damaging impact. I later found out these experiences may have been involved in the development of the chronic daily migraines in addition to the crack on the forehead with the metal T-bar that one summer in Kingston. Apparently, this impact could have weakened the membranes and tiny muscles in the forehead and temple area.

Prior to the onset of the daily headaches, Annie and I were blessed with two healthy boys. Benjamin was born in 1977 and Lucas in 1978. As it is with most parents, I realized the true meaning in my life. I felt on top of the world! Annie and I had always had a close and romantic relationship, and I recall writing songs and short poems to her which she seemed to be always touched by and got a kick out of.

I have fond memories of playing hand hockey with Ben and Luc in the basement, which was covered with a thick, rust-coloured wall-to-wall carpet. We would set up a goal at either end using a stack of books as goal posts, and it would always be the boys against me. The carpet protected our knees as we crawled around trying to score on each other, but it did not protect Luc from getting hit with the homemade ball (newspaper wrapped with duct tape), usually in the head. That would bring the game to a halt!

I would often take the boys to the Clarke on weekends, so we were together. They could watch some TV while I worked on academic endeavours, including completing my BA in psychology and philosophy, which took me thirteen years (one course per year!). It was also important for me to improve my skills at writing detailed clinical and research manuscripts I was engaged in at the time.

My clinical work at the Clarke began with groups of autistic children between the ages of five and nine who had significant difficulties communicating with others. Our program employed "simultaneous communication" (both speaking and signing). At the time, I was struck by the intense, conflicting emotions their parents experienced: warm, caring, loving and sadness, guilt and frustration. I could not imagine how difficult it would be to have an autistic child, as you would have to become hypervigilant. From within this program, I began working with a nine-year-old functionally deaf autistic girl who was blind (Nicola). We met twice a week over the course of six months, and I taught her to sign using the hand-over-hand method. Prior to our working together, she was unable to communicate anything to her parents, but after six months of treatment, with her mom watching from behind a one-way mirror, Nicola developed a vocabulary of more than thirty-three signs that allowed her to express herself to her parents for the first time. Both parents worked hard to use those signs at home, which made all the difference in the world. My work with Nicola and other autistic children, strengthened my compassion for these children and their parents, and my patience for change. This work was detailed in a manuscript published in Child Care Forum (Hunter, D. S. 1983).

I went on to work with a number of youth who were diagnosed with attention deficit and conduct disorder. It was my good fortune to be paired with an amazing co-counsellor, Terryl, who always kept me on my toes. Together, we co-led a few therapeutic day treatment groups with young boys who struggled with various forms of anxiety, depression, and behavioural difficulties. We used a cognitive behavioural approach called "self-instructional training" (Meichenbaum, 1974). Our work was detailed in two follow-up studies published in the Journal of Child and Youth Care (Hunter, D.; et al 1982 and Hunter, D. and Webster, C. 1984). The most interesting results of these studies were that eight years after being in the day treatment groups, these young people remembered all six stages of the self-instructional training as well as every time they were physically restrained by staff! I believed that children who were prone to anger and aggression craved attention, love, and control from the adults in their life. Most often what they received in response was anger, resentment and rejection, a dysfunctional pattern that played out in so many families. Thus, the therapeutic strategies of cognitive therapy were added to my repertoire.

I had many conversations about the impact of staff physically restraining out-of-control youth, many of whom had experienced emotional and physical abuse in their home. One side of the argument was that staff stepping in to take control was continued abuse by the adults in their lives. However, I felt that the loss of control, the anger and aggression, was evidence of "attachment trauma" and a cry for help in controlling overwhelming emotion. In other words, they desperately wanted to be held, to be soothed. I believed that using physical restraint in a calm and caring way was therapeutic and a strategy for repairing attachment trauma. I frequently argued that, from an attachment perspective, these children needed to be held in a calm, reassuring and controlled manner. This was the essence of what professionals called a "corrective experience." I had been involved in well over one hundred physical restraints that employed this method, and it resulted in the development of a more therapeutic relationship with the young people.

It seemed that those staff who struggled to control their own emotions (particularly anger) believed that by making the restraint a punishment (inflicting pain), the youth would be less likely to lose control again. Not only did that not help, but it often made things worse, and that's when people got injured. During my two years working with adolescents at Whitby Psychiatric Hospital, I had been kicked in the face twice and suffered a dislocated elbow because of ineffective restraint techniques being used.

I became a huge fan of all forms of cognitive therapy and engaged in more formal training in this area. The notion of positive self-talk—talking ourselves through problem-solving steps—became an important part of my clinical and personal foundation.

In the Child and Family Studies Centre, Terryl and I taught our day treatment patients using self-instructional training methods. It was a set of five steps to solving a problem (identify the problem, identify possible solutions, make a plan, carry out the plan, and evaluate) at three distinct levels: overt self-guidance (speaking instructions out loud), faded overt self-guidance (whispered instructions) and covert self-guidance (spoken internally). This process was practiced multiple times daily with six children, and the steps were plastered on posters all over the room. Our previous findings triggered my motivation to continue to develop my skills in cognitive therapies and to further investigate the therapeutic use of physical restraints.

CHAPTER 5

THE PAIN ARRIVES

In November 1981, I was set to give a presentation on our follow-up study at a psychology conference in Philadelphia. I had been off work because my sinuses were painful, I could hardly breathe and my ears were starting to ache. Never a good sign. Our GP (Shelly) saw me right away, gave me a prescription for seven days of antibiotics and told me to take decongestants and stay in bed. There was no way I could get on a plane, so I asked my mentor and co-author Chris to do the presentation in my absence. The pain in my face and head became unbearable, so I took some Tylenol 3s and laid on the couch watching television.

I had never felt such pain before. After the antibiotics ran out, I told the doctor that I felt better, but I still had pain across my forehead and behind my eyes. He told me to keep taking the decongestants for another week and let him know how things were going. I was thirty years old and that pain has NEVER gone away.

Shelly, whom I have always loved dearly, was a master diagnostician who wanted to rule out the more serious possibilities. He also thought out loud during his examinations: "Well, it probably has to do with your sinus membranes that can become overly sensitive, but it's best to rule out the more sinister possibilities, so let's get some skull X-rays." Shelly was a little older than Annie and I, with long, black, curly, messy hair. He dressed casually in jeans and a button-down plaid shirt. His voice was low and gravelly, with little emotion in it. It often felt like you were listening to a scientist explain a theory, and he left no stone unturned. When you left Shelly's office, you were always clear about what he thought the problem was, as well as the "differential diagnoses."

I had the X-rays done two days later, just before the holidays. The Thursday before Christmas, Shelly called me at home (he never did that) and said, "Look Don, I don't think this is anything to worry about, but the radiologist who read your X-rays thought that the sella around your pituitary was slightly enlarged, so I want you to see a neurosurgeon just to be sure everything is okay. The earliest appointment we could get was at the end of January. I don't think it's anything to worry about." *Great, thanks Shelly. I won't worry at all for the next six weeks!* I returned to work between Christmas and New Year's, and I was doing a fine job convincing myself that I did in fact have a brain tumour and I didn't have much longer to live! This thinking contributed to the pain, but Sinutab SA gave some relief.

I went into work on a Saturday in early January 1982 to write letters to Annie, Ben and Lucas about how much they meant to me because I was convinced I had a brain tumour and would not likely see the summer! This was such a painful, heart-wrenching experience, but I also felt relief, as I had been thinking about little else since Shelly's phone call. Alone in a day treatment room, I spent more than half the day making sure I shared what I appreciated most about them and my hopes for their future. The tears were unstoppable.

On a positively frigid day in January, I walked into the neurosurgeon's office at Sunnybrook Hospital and sat down. He looked about twenty years old as he held my X-rays up to the light.

"You know the radiologist thought the sella around your pituitary gland looked enlarged, but it looks fine to me. Do you still have the symptoms?"

"Yes. What do you think it might be?" I asked.

He replied, "Well, you may be right about the chronic sinusitis and migraines."

Relieved, I said, "I was prepared to hear that I had a tumour so I am relieved that it may just be chronic sinusitis or migraines."

"What are you taking for the pain?" the doctor asked.

"Sinutab SA, about six a day."

"Well, you might be right, so ask your doctor to try you on some Tylenol 3s for when the Sinutab don't work and check back in six months," he said as he closed my file.

"So it isn't a brain tumour then?" I asked for reassurance.

The doctor smiled and said, "No ... I mean nothing is certain in this business but let me put it this way: I could send you for a CAT scan and even an MRI, but I am 99.5 percent sure there is nothing sinister there. A CAT scan could increase that certainty to 99.6 percent, and an MRI maybe 99.8 percent, but nothing can be 100 percent. You get what I am saying? So, it is your call."

"Well, 99.5 percent certainty is good enough for me, thanks Doc."

I never saw him again.

"What's the next step?" I asked Shelley the next day.

"Well, I will refer you to the pain clinic at Mount Sinai. They have a good reputation. You're booked in two months. In the meantime, how is the pain?"

"Well, on a good day I wake up at about 3 a.m. with a headache about 8/10 on the pain scale," I said, tears forming in my eyes. "I take two Sinutabs and try to get back to sleep, often unsuccessfully. The alarm wakes me at 4:30 a.m., and I struggle to get up and ready to go to work. By the time I've been at work a couple of hours, the pain usually starts to get worse—shooting pains behind the eyes, more right than left, and a throbbing inside my forehead. By the afternoon, the Sinutabs are not working well, so I take two Tylenol 3s. Usually after thirty minutes the pain is down from an 8 to a 4 or 5. I can work like that, but sleeping is becoming a real problem. Sometimes I take two Tylenol 3s at 9 p.m., and by 10:30 I'm not tired and the pain in down to 5. I read but that increases the pain, so I watch TV. By 3 a.m., the pain can climb to 8, and I take two more Tylenols and finally fall asleep about 3:45 a.m. The alarm goes off at 4:30."

Shelly was attentive. "Okay, keep track of the pain and see if the folks at Mount Saini have other suggestions."

In March, I met with the physician at the Mt. Sinai Pain Management Centre and completed ninety minutes of intake questions.

"Well, you have an enormous frontal sinus but nothing sinister that I can see. I believe you have chronic daily headache syndrome, likely with mixed migraine. You say you wake each morning with a low level of pain and as you proceed through each of the many stresses during the day, that pain intensifies?"

Wow! What a surprise! I had dispensed with the Sinutab because they were no longer reducing the pain and stuck to the Tylenol 3s because they at least gave me a couple of hours with the pain under 6. However, by the following Christmas I was taking twelve Tylenol 3s a day and a hypnotic (Imovane) for sleep. I was functioning well considering that the pain level generally hovered between 4 and 6 out of 10 and I had a significant amount of codeine and a hypnotic in my system. I never experienced what I would have considered to be a "high" from the narcotics I was taking—not that was noticeable to me. I simply felt a reduction in the level of pain. I had also trained myself to shift my attention away from my pain to someone else's pain. Through routine daily meditation and cognitive techniques of thought blocking, positive self-talk and self-hypnosis recordings, I actually found that I was able to focus on my clients' stories of pain and suffering better than ever before. Active listening became my greatest skill.

However, in the mid-eighties I realized I was losing what little control I had over the pain. The headaches became more severe, and although I rarely had to take time off work because of the pain, it was having a negative impact in my relationships with family and friends. I tried to maintain a high level of functioning at work and manage the pain at home. I continued with daily meditation to keep myself grounded, as well as developing a positive internal language that helped me hold onto control and kept me focused. For financial reasons, work has always been—and continues to be—the priority.

Shelly supported all my efforts to find alternative treatments, but he was not prepared to prescribe any narcotics stronger than the Tylenol 3s. We tried several other medications, including low dosages of antidepressants and neuroleptics, and he referred me for nerve blocks. I also saw a few chiropractors, physiotherapists, massage therapists, an Ayurvedic physician, a naturopath and someone who did a combination of acupuncture and shiatsu. Apart from acupuncture and shiatsu (which made the pain worse), these practices helped for brief periods. I have always had a needle phobia, so having twenty-two needles stuck in my neck and back before being left alone in a small, dark room for twenty minutes almost triggered a panic attack! The shiatzu therapist explained that my headaches were caused by tight muscle knots in my neck and back, which would require "deep tissue work." The pain from this work was unbearable

"Is it supposed to hurt that much?" I asked.

"Absolutely," he said. "And your experience of the pain confirms that it is a deep tissue problem." I never went back for another shiatzu session!

Nothing I tried lasted except my frustration, fear and hopelessness. I worried every day that the pain would just keep getting worse no matter what I did, that I would soon not be able to work, and we would lose the house. I was terrified that I would have to go on disability and then Annie and the boys would leave me. I wouldn't have blamed them if they did, as I would have left me if I could have! Despite this ever-present "worried view" of the future, I believed in my ability to control my mind, which became my primary strategy in coping with the pain. Daily chanting to stay focused and "covert self-guidance" were the foundation of my strategy. I used two Buddhist chants that held the most meaning for me: the Kanzeon Sutra is quite short, and the Heart of Perfect Wisdom Sutra (also called the Prajna Paramita) is significantly longer. I often recited these two or three times a day to help me focus my attention and connect with my understanding of these chants—that thoughts are simply thoughts, that everything is impermanent, and I need to live every moment I can as fully as I am able.

I had been accepted at York University in 1975 to take one or two courses per year, many of which I took along with my very good friend John Wright (RIP), and I completed my BA in psychology and philosophy. During my final two years at the Clarke, I took on the role of coordinator of children's day treatment, supervising twelve child and youth workers who were responsible for the group treatment of more than thirty children. Just prior to leaving the Clark in 1983, the position of chief child care worker became available. I applied for this position but a person from outside was the successful candidate. One of his first decisions was to remove me as coordinator of day treatment and return me to running groups. In a meeting with him, I shared my disappointment and anger at this decision, as I thought it was not in the best interest of the program. He leaned back in his chair, smiled and with a smug look on his face said, "Let me give you some advice. Don't ever wound a king." As I understood it, I had somehow "wounded" him (the king) by challenging his decision and that I would end up paying for that. One week later, I handed in my resignation.

In 1983, I moved from what was the Clarke Institute of Psychiatry to The Hospital for Sick Children in the newly created position of psychiatric liaison thanks to my friend and colleague Dr. Rod Wachsmuth and Dr. Sue Bradley our Chief Psychiatrist. In this position I was clinically involved in both outpatient and inpatient psychiatry with the unending support from my manager Linda Kostrzewa. During my eight years in this position, I coordinated child and adolescent outpatient groups, co-led inpatient groups, carried out individual and family therapy, was an active part of the nursing management team, provided clinical supervision to frontline nurses as well as child and youth counsellors, and co-facilitated a multidisciplinary supervisory group for therapists who were leading therapy groups for youth. I did all this with another amazing mentor, Dr. Harvey Armstrong. I was using all my clinical skills with patients and myself!

In 1986, I began in a part-time clinical master's program at McMaster University in health sciences (MHSc). I completed this program in 1989. My thesis for my masters involved a retrospective study on the co-incidence of birthdays and psychiatric admissions of adolescents within thirty days pre or post their birthday. My thesis proposal was a hard sell to my advisor, Dr. Gina Browne at McMaster University. However, after explaining my rationale for choosing this topic, she provided her full support. The results of this study were eventually published in the Journal of Child and Youth Care (Hunter, Don S. (1995).

The results supported the hypothesis that significantly more young people would be admitted to our psychiatric unit within thirty days pre or post their birthday than any other time of the year. Although this study has never been replicated, we continue to see many young people admitted to our facility within that time frame.

It remains my perspective that approaching birthdays are often stressful as people, young and old, reflect on the previous year. If it had been a particularly difficult year, there can be many worries about how the next year will pan out. Worries about past, present and future can weigh most heavily just before or just after one's birthday! When I defended my thesis, the committee asked the question, "So what is the clinical relevance of your findings?" My response was brief: "Parents, teachers, therapists and physicians need to be aware of the likelihood of increased stress and anxiety as birthdays approach and as they fade. Extra kindness and support may help to prevent a crisis!" That response seemed acceptable.

I was so fortunate to have been a part of such a rich clinical experience during those years. I attended a Cape Cod Institute for advanced cognitive-behavioural training and secured hour for hour supervision from some of the most experienced psychiatrists at the hospital for my individual, family, and group work in both inpatient and outpatient psychiatry. I was confident and excited about my work, and I was determined to not allow the pain and medications interfere.

During the late-eighties, I spent my summer vacation time at a private children's camp. Annie was a nurse there, which allowed Ben and Luc to attend camp, and I eventually took on the role as a program lead. Our abode was the health centre, and we had constant contact with the camp physicians, so I shared my struggles with them. One of these doctors (Lorne) was working with chronic pain using nerve blocks and suggested I consider trying it. Once back in the city, I met with Lorne and shared a brief written story of my experiences since the pain began. His response was to ask, "Do you think you are depressed?"

"Well, having this pain all the time is depressing," I said with a smile, "but I don't believe it is a 'clinical depression.' Besides, I have strategies for coping."

Regardless, Lorne put me on a trial of low-dose antidepressants along with weekly nerve blocks—ten or so injections of a cortisone and novocaine mix which essentially froze the nerves where I experienced the most pain (forehead and temples). The ten to twelve hours that the freezing lasted was the only time I had without pain, but was it worth it to have those few hours of relief given the cost? I had the blocks weekly for about three months and then stopped. I tried the antidepressants, but they did not seem to help much, and I eventually just drifted away from this whole process.

I had spoken to Shelly about the increasing buzzing, ringing and wind blowing in my ears that always got worse at night. I remember him saying, "There is no cure for tinnitus. The only treatment for it is to listen to something louder than it is." I was already listening to music, self-hypnosis recordings and watching movies at night to distract from the pain, so now I would just crank up the volume to drown out the tinnitus! As is always the case, we become accustomed to a broad range of things, and as we adapt, such things have less of an impact. I remember thinking about the first five years of my life growing up with the powerful sounds of trains going by my house and how it became less noticeable and, in fact, almost comforting. The tinnitus was never comforting, but the impact weakened significantly over time.

In 1987, I was approached to participate in training with a self-help organization called Bereaved Families of Ontario (BFO). This involved eight full Saturdays led by two seasoned clinicians, David Wright and Rheba Adolph, along with the BFO program staff. All BFO's group facilitators had experienced the death of a child or sibling, participated in the mutual self-help groups that the organization facilitated and then became group facilitators themselves. This experience was both life-changing and life-confirming for me. That first Saturday of training began with all twelve members sharing their tragic, painful stories of loss. As I listened to their stories, I dreaded the moment when I would have to share my own, as I had no idea what I would share. I was unsure of why I had agreed to volunteer for this but, as each painful and tragic story of loss unfolded, I found my memory resurrecting my experiences with loss. When it came to my turn to share why I was there, I wiped the tears from my eyes and informed the group how deeply moved I was to hear their stories of loss and that I could never imagine their grief. I simply shared that one thing I had learned from that day was how important it is to be able to share the experience of loss and how much it resonates with everyone.

The following week was a struggle, as I would find myself recalling some of the painful stories I had listened to. This triggered my own connection with loss, causing me to revisit my core beliefs about death and dying while carrying out my clinical work. I came to realize this was yet another struggle that would ultimately enhance my clinical skills and my compassion for the suffering of others.

Just prior to leaving The Hospital for Sick Kids in 1990, I had started a small, part-time private practice and accepted a part-time teaching contract at Ryerson University in the child and youth counsellor program. Having graduated from the Master's in Health Sciences program at McMaster University, an amazing clinical program, this move into teaching made sense. The daily pain continued to get worse, and my response was to "do" more! I volunteered to co-facilitate groups at BFO and joined their professional advisory committee, which included co-facilitating two-day grief workshops.

Annie kept herself busy, taking on various roles with television production companies. Both of us were becoming more focused on work, and the boys, who were well into adolescence, each had their own joys and struggles. But Annie and I had little time to devote to the "us" part of our relationship. It was at this time that the owners of the summer camp (Tamarack) we had been involved in since 1985 offered me a co-director position, which I accepted. This provided me with a steady income, office space and required a minimal time commitment between September and May each year. With the pain climbing yet again, I had to increase the dosages of the narcotics to get the relief I needed to work. I found that even when I was off work and stress was low, the pain level did not change.

My volunteer time with BFO was both painful and inspirational, touching my soul and adding greatly to the strength of my compassion, which became the foundation of all my work and my family life. I began co-facilitating parent mutual support groups that were led by a bereaved, volunteer parent and a professional advisor for parents who had lost children due to illness, suicide, and murder—all profoundly painful experiences and reinforcing of one's priorities in life. During the initial training in 1988, I was so moved by the powerful personal experiences people shared, that I needed to write about it, which resulted in a song. As I made my way through that first mutual support group for parents, the song I had written after that training seemed to fit for this group. I present this here because it captures the essence of this experience.

FOREVER YOURS

I look around me and I see tired faces,
I see that there's pain that goes straight through the heart.
And I see that the love for the life that's been lost,
Is so great no one else can imagine the cost.
I try to imagine the pain that you're feeling,
I try to imagine your loss as my own.
I try to imagine myself in your place,
But that's just too painful for me.
You talk about things that make me feel fearful,
That make me step back and take stock of my life.
At times it still scares me, what drew me to you,
But I know I'm a better person because of you.
I wish I could give you back the life that you lost,

I wish I could take away all your pain.
And I wish I could turn back the hands of time,
But that's impossible, I know.

And for you, that pain in your life is still there,
All the talk and the sharing can't take that away.

But today it seems different, life has new meaning,
Today I can hear laughter, that's right from your heart.

I wish I could give you back the life that you lost,
I wish I could take away all your pain,
And I wish I could turn back the hands of time,
But that's impossible, I know.

Think about life and how it is at this moment.
Think about the joy life can bring to you.
In today there's a hope for a brighter tomorrow,
A hope from that love, forever yours.

(10.10.88)

Somehow, I managed to drum up the courage to bring my guitar and share the song with the group during our last session. Tearful expressions of sadness and resonance confirmed that singing this song was cathartic—for everyone. One of our group members approached me after group and asked if I would play that song for a support group he belonged to at his place of worship. That group also found that the lyrics resonated with them.

The second group I had the honour of co-facilitating was a young adult group. Each participant had lost a parent, brother or sister. Once again, such a profound experience led to yet another song, which was a way for me to share the essence of what I received from them.

Someone's Missing

So, this is what love is about,
The sense of loss and emptiness inside.
We pay for our loving with our pain,
There is no place anyone can hide.

Chronic Pain: My Journey

What sense can be made of this tragedy?
What reason can justify my pain?
Someone show me the way out of here,
I fear that I am going insane.
I want to touch you just one more time,
Want to feel you close to me.
Some say, "Forget, it it's over now,"
But it's only beginning for me.

Someone in here is missing, someone so many people loved.
Someone isn't here who is needed so. Who will help us now?
Who will help us now?

It's only right to be crying, only right to feel afraid.
The only thing that keeps us going,
Is the hope that they will walk back through that door,
While knowing we won't see them anymore.

I could not stay, it was too painful for me, to watch you suffer so.
It hurts to think about it now, I just can't let you go.
My life lost all its meaning the day you went away.
All you left are my memories and I'm terrified they will not stay.
I miss your smile, I miss your laughter, I
miss the way you cared for me.
No one knew just what we had. And what we had, no one could see.
Because it belonged to you and to me.

It's hard to face what happened, hard to look life in the eye.
Tough to get up and get your feet back on the ground,
Knowing that an important part of you is gone.
It often feels like we're just floating, like it's all quite unreal.
No one else knows what it's like.
Can they see the pain I feel inside?
Can they feel the pain I try to hide?

I turn around and it's all so confusing,
Nothing makes sense anymore.

So many feelings I can't explain, I just walk out the door.
I know that there will come a time,
When things will be clearer to me,
But, for now, I'll let these feelings just flow over me.

(06.06.91)

I struggled with the daily pain in my head throughout this time, but that pain paled significantly in the presence of those who were grieving the loss of a loved one. I was desperately focused on organizing what I was learning through experience in these groups in a way that facilitated my own understanding and growth as a clinician—and as a person. After all, it is all connected and intertwined!

I continued my daily meditations and cognitive behavioural strategies, and I decided I would work on my self-hypnosis program. I had taken a course on hypnosis during my time at the Clarke Institute, so I connected with a wonderful psychiatrist, Adam Stein, who used hypnosis in managing chronic pain. I had about twelve sessions with him, and he recorded each session on cassette tapes I could listen to between sessions. I found his South African accent to be very soothing! This experience was valuable, and I developed my own recordings which combined gentle music and the sounds of the ocean with my voice delivering the guided meditations for pain relief.

Self-hypnosis became part of my daily practice, and along with meditation, was the key component that kept me sane and able to focus on my work and continue to learn and grow my clinical skills. Unfortunately, the pain continued to worsen. I awoke each morning with pounding in my head and went to bed each night with sharp stabbing pains in my temples and behind my eyes. The

Tylenol 3s I was taking were becoming less effective. My family and social life paid a heavy price, as most of my time at home was in bed, taking the multiple medications and watching movies as a distraction. There were more frequent visits to Sunnybrook Emergency Department when the pain would become unbearable. In those moments, all I wanted to do was ram my head into a wall. The ER doctors gave me an Ativan (an antianxiety medication) and ran a Toradol drip (a non-narcotic analgesic). After about an hour, the pain would drop from 9 down to 7, which was enough for me to return home to bed.

At a time when I could not imagine my daily struggle getting worse, things really got quite dark!

CHAPTER 6

INTO THE ABYSS

Shelly had referred me to a pain clinic where I tried a variety of medications and procedures including migraine medication (Zomig, Imitrex), morphine, Halcion, Dilaudid, fentanyl, amitriptyline, nerve blocks, Botox, etc. I vomited multiple times a day during the first few weeks on the fentanyl patches (25 mcg every forty-eight hours to start), and I realized this was a very powerful narcotic! However, the vomiting stopped, and the pain level dropped to 3 out of 10, so I was quite joyful for the next few months. I felt more in control, more engaged in my family and friend relationships, and I had so much more hope. These positive effects began to wear off and increases in dosage happened at the three- and six-month mark.

Within the first year of using the fentanyl, I had increased to 100 mcg every forty-eight hours. Most medications began with promise and hope, as did all the "alternative" therapies. Initially, each new medication brought down the pain by at least 3 points. However, within no time the pain was back up again so we had to increase the dose or frequency. The self-hypnosis and meditation allowed me to hold onto my focus on all that was good in my life, particularly when the pain would hit 9 and 10. I would spend almost all my time at home in bed alternating heat and ice, chanting, listening to hypnosis tapes and watching movies through the nights, as I could not sleep for long before the pain woke me. Even with high doses of hypnotic medications, I would be woken with that all too familiar stabbing pain every couple of hours.

We eventually switched from Imovane to Triazolam, which helped me sleep and dropped the pain level to between 4 and 7 out of 10; I had become accustomed to functioning well at that level. The self-hypnosis recordings, meditation and chanting continued to be a daily ritual in my attempts to "train my brain" to control the pain. I even listened to one during lunch breaks at work or before teaching a class. Frequent self-hypnotic sessions helped me manage the pain and become a more compassionate therapist with an ever-broadening repertoire of strategies and techniques to help clients—and myself.

I became increasingly able to shift my focus away from my pain and towards the physical and emotional pain of others. I continued with my private practice and volunteering with BFO, co-facilitating groups and grief workshops. I also accepted a position as co-director of a private summer camp (Camp Tamarack) that we had been involved with for numerous summers. These experiences were immensely helpful in strengthening my belief in the therapeutic value of helping others of any age, and it helped me maintain my priorities in life.

I needed to stay busy, and to keep learning and growing as a clinician. My work became my escape from the pain, and I accepted another part-time position as manager of school services for Earlscourt Child and Family Centre. I had the privilege of supervising four amazing child and youth counsellors who carried out a variety of school programs in thirteen elementary schools in the west end of Toronto. We coordinated the development and implementation of classroom presentations on anti-bullying, valuing pro-social behaviour and problem-solving, and we established a variety of peer support groups. The instances of bullying in all our schools dropped significantly. My eighteen months there was another positive clinical experience, but I felt that I had bitten off more than I could chew!

At home, I focused on my relationship with my boys, as I reminded myself daily that they needed my involvement and participation in their lives. However, managing the pain, work and my relationship with the boys left Annie sort of in the background, which took an increasing toll on our relationship. The narcotics and hypnotics had an enormous impact on my libido, making intimacy difficult. I searched for something—anything! —that would take this pain away, and this obsessive search led me down some dark paths. Thoughts of my life ending would frequently come into my awareness as a vague wish to bring an end to the pain. I never seriously considered suicide, but I entertained many different scenarios about ways I could be killed—drive-by shooting, carjacking, trying to stop a fight and getting killed. This wish was front and centre in my mind for far too long, so I chanted to refocus, shifting away from negative thoughts, and focusing on being mindful of the present moment. The daily use of the coping strategies, particularly the deep breathing, meditation, and positive self-talk, developed into a habit of reminding myself to stay in the present moment. This was so important for my clinical work, my teaching, and my personal relationships.

In the summer of 1994, my best friend Elton took his own life. Elton, his wife Barb and their amazing children, Vanessa, Tristan, Rebecca and Mary, have always been a loving part of our family. I was at camp when I received a call from Annie to tell me the terrible news. I broke down immediately. I felt such intense pain, and my stomach and chest tightened as if in a vice. I ran to my cabin, collapsed on the bed, and screamed the things I wanted to say to him into a pillow as an intense sense of loss numbed me. I was angry that he didn't reach out and that he would make such a drastic choice. I knew he was struggling, and after a visit, we would always hug and I would say, "If you need anything, we are here." He would simply respond with, "I know." I believe that when depression gains power and control, it convinces the host that they are nothing but a burden and everyone would be better off without them—often financially as well. I have come to call this "depression's delusion" because my experience with families who have lost a member to suicide is that they are never "better off"! I have memories of Elton come back to me at some point every day, and when I am struggling with choices, I always ask for his input!

I was surprised that such a loss did not make the pain in my head worse. This was also true when my younger brother Greg died in 2004, my dad in 2009 and my mom in 2012. It became apparent that the core of the chronic pain I experience daily exists independent of emotional stress and strain; it waxes and wanes no matter what happens. My daily practice of relaxing, calming, accepting, and focusing meditations established a pattern of responding to daily stressful experiences from a state of relaxed calm. I would notice many times a day that my body was engaged in deep diaphragmatic breathing. I would recite a chant or mantra to shift attention away from the pain, enabling me to focus. I continued to utilize the two primary chants I have used for many years—the Kanzeon Sutra and the Prajna Paramita—sometimes multiple times a day. If the pain rose above a 6/10 when I was driving, I would use these chants to remain mindful of my driving. I had stopped listening to the radio or music while driving because I needed to pay attention to the road.

In 2000, I lost my contract with the summer camp and with Bereaved Families of Ontario where I had been the clinical consultant since 1995. I also decided to stop teaching at Ryerson. Although I loved the actual teaching, marking student papers and dealing with complex students was taking far too much of my time. I secured a position as program director for Gilda's Club Toronto, a cancer support organization, which was scheduled to open in March 2001. I interviewed with their selection committee, which included the executive director (I'll call her Mya), the chair of the board of directors and one other member of the board—all such kind and compassionate people. After sharing the training and experience I believed qualified me for the position, I was asked to tell them a joke. This caught me totally off guard. Telling jokes has never been a strength, however, I did offer to sing them a song, "Signifying Monkey," a humorous song about a monkey, a lion and an elephant. Despite my off-key voice, they seemed impressed that I would do that!

I had enormous respect for Mya, and I had a transforming experience when we spent seven days together training at the Gilda's Club in New York. The training involved people sharing painful experiences about living with and in proximity to cancer. The old fire hall in downtown Toronto was the Gilda's Club Toronto headquarters, and it was under renovations. We began developing training programs for volunteers, as well as the range of services we would offer to our clients. I hired a hard-working young woman (I'll call her Lena) I worked with at Bereaved Families of Ontario to help with the program development.

Things seemed to be going along as planned, but I became concerned when I had the feeling that something was happening behind my back between Lena and Mya. Over the next three months, my work in training volunteers was criticized and Mya gave me a letter indicating that I needed to "improve" how I trained the volunteers if I were to remain in this position. This was a real shock, as I felt the training sessions were going well and I had already started facilitating a support group. I struggled with daily migraines, but feedback from participants indicated I was providing a solid training experience for our volunteers and a strong, supportive group for clients, so I was confused.

The day before my six-month probation period was up, I was in my office around 7:30 a.m. when I heard footsteps coming up the stairs. It gave me an uneasy feeling. Mya and the chair of the board walked into my office and informed me that they had decided I was not the right person for this position. I was immediately escorted out of the building and told that I could make arrangements to pick up my belongings the following morning. When I arrived the following morning, there were boxes at the foot of the staircase packed with my belongings and, as Mya said goodbye, I caught a glimpse of my assistant Lena moving things into my former office. Another uneasy feeling washed over me. *There's something fishy going on here!* I thought.

When I was going through my box of files at home, I noticed that all the files regarding Gilda's Club, including my program of volunteer training and files on program development, were gone, which I had expected. However, there was an unmarked folder which contained a copy of a long letter from Lena to Mya outlining how incompetent I was for the program director position and how she should be the one in that position! Et tu, Brute? I had stayed in touch with one of our volunteers over the following few months through emails, and she informed me that Lena, who had taken over as program director, was also let go. I told her about the letter I had found, and she was not surprised that Lena had orchestrated my dismissal. I recall ending this email by saying that she had stabbed me in the back and somehow this email exchange landed in Mya's email box as well. She emailed me to say that she had also been stabbed in the back. Interesting outcome!

Needless to say, this experience did nothing to ease the pain in my head. I still had my small private practice where I worked with clients in their homes while continuing my search for steady employment. After several interviews, I accepted a full-time counselling position with East Metro Youth Services (EMYS) to provide individual, group and family counselling in Scarborough. I continued with my daily mindful practices along with a powerful combination of medications. My work remained my top priority—*I can't give in to this pain!* My work with EMYS was incredibly satisfying in so many ways. Although it has always been my clinical work with clients and patients that is most rewarding, the colleagues I had the privilege of working alongside at EMYS were among the most compassionate, committed, and dedicated professionals I had encountered.

In 2001, I was also fortunate to be offered a position as a consultant on a television competition program called *Canadian Idol*, which was produced by Insight Productions. In this position I was responsible for providing emotional and psychological support to the competitors. This show ran for six seasons, and it was an amazing experience for me as I had the distinct honour of working with a great production team as well as hundreds of young people from across Canada who competed each May for the top twenty spots. Each four-month season provided me with the opportunity to work with these young performers for approximately ten hours a week, that time spent before and during each show. I connected with young people who had a dream they had been chasing for a long time, and this gave me a perspective on youth I had been missing. These young people struggled with anxieties and had conflicted relationships just like the youth I worked with in therapy. The important difference was that the youth involved with *Canadian Idol* were highly motivated and had a passion and clear goals they were working towards. They were like a breath of fresh air!

I committed to this work despite my daily struggle with pain. I had to find ways to carry out my responsibilities, so I would spend twenty to thirty minutes in my car, in my quiet space, listening to self-hypnosis recordings before entering the venue to connect with the production team and the competitors. This ritual was absolutely essential for me to be able to focus on others and their experiences with anxiety and stress.

I had also rekindled my connection with SickKids Hospital by accepting a part-time position with the psychiatry department working in the crisis and eating disorder programs. When I decided to leave EMYS in 2005, I accepted a full-time position at SickKids and secured an office in the community for my private practice. I had become a member of the Ontario Association of Social

Workers and Registered Social Service Workers (OASWSSW) as a Registered Social Worker (RSW).

When I was hired at that time, the only position open was for a child and youth counsellor within the psychiatry inpatient program. I accepted this position with the understanding that I could apply for any social work positions that became available. Such a position became available in our eating disorders day program, and I was interviewed, but it did not pan out. I have applied for four other social work positions at SickKids over the past twenty years and never received any response whatsoever!

I have concluded that there are three potential explanations why. First, the hospital is funded for specific positions with specific qualifications. Social workers must have graduated from an accredited Master's in Social Work (MSW) program; therefore, my clinical Master's in Health Sciences (MHSc) would not qualify. The second possibility is that my senior colleagues did not believe that I possessed the clinical expertise to fulfill the requirements of the position. The third possibility is that my senior colleagues did not like me personally (this is the one that hurt the most).

I chose to believe the first scenario, so I contacted the director of the social work program at a local university and arranged for a meeting. I asked her about the requirements to complete the master's program in social work given that I already had a master's in health sciences. She explained that it would take a year but then asked why I would take that path when I already had the clinical skills and experience at above a master's requirements. We talked about the various PhD programs in social work, as she believed that would be a better option, but this was not a possibility financially. So, I remained in the child and youth counsellor position and maintained my focus on my clinical work at the hospital and my private practice as an RSW.

I redoubled my determination and commitment to learning therapeutic modalities that were considered best practices. This included advanced cognitive behavioural therapy, attending intensive training workshops in narrative therapy with Michael White, and completing an advanced externship in brief and narrative therapy. Neurolinguistic programing, eye movement desensitization and reprocessing, and hypnotherapy certifications added to my growing repertoire of therapeutic skills. On the side, I was reading everything I could find regarding neuroplasticity, and living with and managing chronic pain.

I was concerned about my visits to Sunnybrook Emergency when the pain reached 9 or 10, and it finally dawned on me that sitting there for hours was a bad idea because it wasn't helping! I had consulted with several different "pain experts" who suggested I would benefit from having a separate narcotic to treat what they called "breakthrough pain" (when the pain would "breakthrough" the daily dose of fentanyl). I thought this would be far better than more visits to the emergency room. The "breakthrough" medications varied between Dilaudid, Hydromorphone and OxyContin. All started out being very helpful but contributed to my dependence on the narcotics for pain relief, at increased dosages.

I had done some reading about massage techniques in addition to essential oils in treating migraines, and I, thankfully, found Sharon, who connected me with Young Living Essential Oils. She started each day with a few drops of therapeutic grade frankincense oil and one drop of peppermint in a shot of red juice, claiming she felt more energized and ready for her day. Since that time, I start every day with five drops of therapeutic grade frankincense oil and a drop of peppermint in a shot of milk or juice. Having continued this practice now for over fifteen years, I believe that this has had a therapeutic effect on my internal organs and immune system. Given my daily use of a variety of pain medications, at high doses, we were always concerned with my liver and kidney functioning, but the routine testing has always been within normal limits. Although I don't have scientific evidence to support this, the way I feel reinforces the power of my belief in the benefits of this practice.

During this time, Shane, my pain doctor, referred me to a specialist in a pain clinic at Sunnybrook Hospital who was investigating a technique for treating chronic pain called rhizolysis. He explained that my brain was receiving pain signals from the nerves in my back even though there may not be any "real pain," and my brain had been wired to just keep receiving these phantom pain signals. So, the procedure was to cauterize the specific nerves responsible so no pain signals reached the brain, which would allow my brain to "re-program" itself. The cauterized nerves would regenerate eventually, and the expectation was that the brain should have re-programmed itself by then. The results of this experience included a couple of months of annoying pain at the surgical sight, frustration that it didn't work and increased loss of hope that I would find anything that would take the pain away.

After Shane moved out west in 2006, his colleague Jan, who I had known since starting with Shane, agreed to take over. Jan was always the one who administered the sedative before I had the nerve block injections. At that time, I was on 150 mcg of fentanyl every forty-eight hours, OxyContin for breakthrough pain, and 75 mg of Triazolam to help with sleep. We were always concerned with dependency and addiction, and Jan was strict in prescribing and monitoring the medications. He always reminded me that the goal was to get off the narcotics, as he believed they were making the pain worse. I was resistant to this idea primarily out of fear of the increased pain I would experience and that I would end up losing everything.

Eventually it became clear that I was dependent on the narcotics for pain relief and that I was not chasing any high from the medications. The "experts" had convinced me that the body uses the narcotics to treat the pain, not get me high. There was always a large quantity of narcotic medications within reach on my bedside table, but I was usually able to resist the temptation to take more than was prescribed. I believed I was "dependent," not "addicted" (a solid rationalization!). I manipulated my use of the medications by adding heat to the fentanyl patches during the last few hours before I could put a new patch on. I would also split up the dose of Triazolam to see if it would keep the pain under 7 out of 10. This manipulation seemed to be helpful, as it was administering the medication differently, but this beneficial effect also wore off with time, like everything else.

It became more and more difficult to accept that the pain might never go away, and I was also becoming more depressed about what this journey with the pain had cost me in my family and social life. If I was not at work, teaching or in training, I was home in bed. When I attended social events, it was never for more than a few hours before I would have to excuse myself so I could lay down and engage in my routine for getting through the really, painful times. This included a dark, quiet room, self-hypnosis recordings, a tight band around my head, and cold or hot packs. What a life! Making it through the twelve-hour shifts at the hospital was becoming increasingly difficult, particularly the night shifts, as I have never been able to sleep where I work. By the tenth hour (about 5:30 a.m.), my head would be pounding, there would be sharp pain behind my eyes, and I was exhausted. I was using up all my sick time and eventually asked Jan to write a letter to support my request to be taken off the night shift. Much to our dismay, the "accommodation committee" rejected the recommendation, and this resulted in me using all my sick time every month. Jan then decided to write a more forceful letter to the committee. This time they accepted the recommendation to eliminate night shifts and allowed me to use vacation time if I had to be off work due to the pain and had no sick time left. This was a big win and a huge relief.

I thought about Annie every day, and I felt sorry for the changes that had occurred in our lives. We weren't able to regain the amazing romantic relationship we had, and I wanted to apologize, but I believed it would only make things worse. From my perspective, I assumed that she felt helpless, as there was nothing she could do to help me with the pain. She had to do virtually everything around the house. We avoided conversations about what we were both going through—*What would be the point?* The changes in our relationship were the most painful thing for me because of how much I enjoyed helping and how much I loved the romantic moments in our life—the emotional poems, a few songs, the daily playfulness, the laughter. I desperately wanted it back. During one of these dark, painful experiences I somehow managed to get some thoughts on paper about the love of my life.

I Am So Sorry, Annie

I have heard the phrase "Love means never having to say you are sorry," but I feel such powerful remorse & regret that you deserve a sincere apology.

I feel so sorry that, when the pain came on, I turned to a never-ending search for a medication to take the pain away. I didn't realize I would have to live with some degree of pain for the rest of my life, so I continued to try increasingly potent medications. They were all helpful in reducing the pain initially, but looking back, I can see that they ended up making the pain worse.

I feel so sorry that I became less and less available to you, our boys and our friends. That the combination of the pain and the medications led to a significant reduction in my more romantic and playful side. That we lost that closeness we had for so many years.

I feel so sorry that I became so self-centred and focused on my work and managing the pain that I neglected my role as a loving and caring partner.

I feel so sorry that I placed work and managing the pain in first and second place when you and the boys should have always come first.

Chronic Pain: My Journey

I thought about this catch 22 I was in, and I was conscious of the choices I felt I had to make. I regretted these choices, but I couldn't figure it out and I couldn't talk about it even though I thought about our relationship every single day. Not knowing what to do next and feeling stuck always pulled me back into the pain.

I let you down! I was not strong enough to change things.

I became so unattractive—I didn't even want to spend time with me!

I became aware of how hard it is to live with someone with chronic pain. There is absolutely nothing attractive about that, and it must have been painful to realize there's nothing you could do to make the pain go away.

I feel so sorry that I don't share with you, each and every day, how deeply I love you. I am afraid of triggering feelings of sympathy and guilt, and I have already put you through enough.

I am so sorry that the last thirty years have not been what we once dreamed of for our future.

I am so sorry that other people's stories and pain have been the thing that helps me to not give in to the pain I experience.

I keep trying to develop better control over this pain so I can enjoy more and more of my life and care for you in the way you deserve.

And I will keep trying as long as I live.

You have no idea how much I have appreciated every day that you have stayed beside me. You deserve so much more.

XXOO

CHAPTER 7

CLIMBING OUT

In January 2010, I was dangerously close to the end of my rope. I'd spent too many nights meditating, chanting, and praying to try and relieve the pain. My final prayer was always, "Please God, take my soul before I wake," a variation of the prayer "Now I Lay Me Down to Sleep" I repeated every night as a child.

Those close to me were aware that the pain was getting worse, and I was becoming more distant. Judi and Chaim, who are very close friends and had significant experience in the field of addictions, were incredibly loving and supportive. They encouraged me to see a physician with expertise in this area, as they felt the narcotics I had been taking were making things worse. I met with this doctor, who was engaging and supportive, and who concurred that I needed to come off all the narcotics so the level of pain could be re-evaluated. Jan had been encouraging me to come off the narcotics for a long time, so after several conversations with Annie and some close friends, I entered the medical withdrawal unit at CAMH for seven days.

This was a most difficult process, but it was cleansing, inspiring and spiritual, to say the least. I intensified my meditation and use of self-hypnosis recordings despite the pain, nausea and vomiting from withdrawal. I even attempted painting, which I enjoyed, but the results reinforced my significant lack of talent and skill! The pain and anguish of those first three days gave way to a realization of the negative impact of long-term narcotic use to treat chronic pain; It eventually just makes everything worse. I also realized how important the love of family and friends is when taking on such a monumental task. I had imaginary visits from the family members I had lost, including Elton. The support and wisdom they shared, I understood as my own but hearing it in their voices was more powerful.

It felt like a form of rebirth, and I was a little on the "manic" side of things for a few weeks. I was overly excited about the prospect of establishing better control over the pain and very hopeful that my relationships would improve. I left hospital with a prescription for Gabapentin (a non-narcotic), as the medical folks felt this should be helpful. The throbbing in my temples and the frequent lightning strikes behind the eyes—especially when there were significant shifts in weather conditions—still plagued me, but it seemed somehow more manageable and not as intense. As I continued with the daily practices that helped me cope, regular changes in weather increased the intensity of the pain. I noticed a significant shift in my energy level and ability to engage and focus at work. Several colleagues had noticed a difference in me and thought I seemed "more alive." This made me realize that, despite my counselling skills, I was obviously struggling prior to staying at CAMH. Memories of intense pain during a shift and having to take an hour to put a cold pack on my head and listen to a guided meditation so I could refocus came back to me.

In the absence of narcotics, I was functioning better in my work but slipping back into the cycle of focusing intensely on my daily clinical work rather than my pain, until I got home. Then I went to bed to watch movies, listen to my hypnosis recordings, apply ice packs and sleep when I could. I stopped the Gabapentin, as it did not help much, and alternated between Tylenol Extra Strength, Advil, and Aleve. I was not feeling particularly happy even though I experienced moments of joy with family and friends. Although these times didn't last long, I felt far better than before.

Chronic Pain: My Journey

When I got home from the medical withdrawal unit, Annie asked if the pain was better.

"It won't work if you lie to me!" she said.

I decided it would have been overwhelming for her if I were to share when the pain was intense and all those thoughts about not wanting to keep fighting and not having much hope! I chose to be vague when sharing anything about the pain rather than lying.

"Ah, it's been worse…"

"I'm okay…"

"It's a bit distracting…"

"I'm working on it…"

And so on. I purposely held back on the deeper thoughts because I was afraid of giving them more power by actually saying them out loud. It is a dilemma because I encourage patients and clients to do the opposite and share their struggles with troublesome thoughts and emotions openly because it actually weakens them. However, the fear of the negative impact on others has always been too powerful for me to stand against.

I would try to reason with myself. *Look, you advise kids and parents to open up with each other, to share their pain and to be honest. You have seen this help their relationships so why can't you do the same?* However, most of the folks I worked with in the hospital and privately had a clear direction they could take to resolve the problems. When it comes to chronic pain (as well as other chronic conditions), there is no path that can lead to resolution, and because this is the reality, I believed that sharing all the negative thoughts and feelings with those I love would burden them. *What are they supposed to do with that information?* I thought. Besides, I always believed that Annie was well aware when the pain was very bad, so I didn't need to go on and on about it. When there is no solution in sight, repeated sharing of the same problem leaves others feeling frustrated, helpless, and hopeless.

I read as much as I could about neuroplasticity, the neurology of chronic pain, and potential migraine solutions. I took on a year of training in neurolinguistic programming (NLP) and earned a certificate as an NLP practitioner. This was another amazing program that added significantly to my clinical skills and the use of my mind to develop better control over how I responded to the pain. It was a maintenance program that provided additional positive self-talk to help me remain mindful and feel more grounded.

I had climbed out of a rut but still had a long way to go. I had read a lot about the use of medical cannabis in treating a wide range of illnesses, including chronic pain. After conversations with Jan about how this may help me to sleep, improve my mood and hopefully decrease the need for the over-the-counter analgesics, he agreed to make the referral. After a year of experimenting with medical cannabis that contained high levels of cannabidiol (CBD) and low levels of tetrahydrocannabinol (THC), I could finally enjoy social and family activities more and sleep a little better, but I still had to take the analgesics during the day to drop the pain level, and at night to get to sleep. I quickly moved from baking edible cannabis products to the far simpler CBD 1:1 oil, which I sprayed into my mouth as needed. My experience was that, within twenty to thirty minutes I was in a better mood and able to shift away from the pain and focus on more pleasant activities—walking our dog, having a conversation with Annie or the boys, cleaning, and planning get-togethers.

Even still, I was most often in bed after work and spent a great deal of time reading and learning about a range of psychotherapeutic modalities. This always helped to keep me feeling sharp, on my toes and focused on listening to other people's stories of pain and struggling in their lives. Learning new and different strategies added to my "toolkit" of techniques for my clients and for myself. Financially, the work was critical— the bills still had to be paid! It was also an important way to retain purpose in my career. I became quite fearful of not being able to work every day. I needed to develop other endeavours to generate meaning in my life beyond the pain, above the pain, below the pain or wherever the pain is less intense.

There are a few important things I do in my mind and body every day. Each morning, sitting on the edge of the bed, I notice the pain in my lower back (spinal stenosis and osteoarthritis). As I take a few deep, slow breaths, I arch my back gently and focus my attention on how that reduces that pain. I then move to my yoga mat, continuing the deep breathing, and complete a series of gentle stretches for by lower back and legs, which allows me to walk without too much pain. I silently chant the Prajnaparamita and Kanzeon Sutras and repeat the four "duties" in Jiulong Baguazhang (Bagua): honesty with myself and others; humility in thought, word and deed; patience and serving others according to their needs; and sincerity is the foundation of my every action and has also become a chant. This process takes between ten and twenty minutes.

I then spend ten to twenty minutes practicing a series of postures and actions from Bagua called the Daoyin (Appendix A), which also helps my muscles and joints to loosen. Bagua is often referred to as an "internal martial art," which I understand to mean that every movement comes from inside the body and mind, so they need to be trained together. From my perspective, the essence of mindfulness is focused attention on the muscles that move the body and the balanced use of force. Through this morning routine, I am aware of the pain in my head but work to maintain my focus on what is happening in the rest of my body and, as often as I can do this, the pain intensity decreases.

Most nights remain a struggle, as I can feel myself giving in to the constant noise in my ears, which often sounds like a field of a million crickets all rubbing their legs at the same time, the stabbing pain behind my eyes and the alternating throbbing in my temples. That fear that I will slip into that deep, dark rabbit hole where helplessness and hopelessness reside comes into awareness again.

Fuck, I can't do this again! I can't focus on this …
Breathe … let it go.

CHAPTER 8

ROUTINES AND RITUALS

Preventing myself from slipping into this dark place is always incredibly difficult! It is hard to keep moving forward, to engage in life as much as possible despite the pain, but so many people do so with more challenges than I face. That notion, along with spending time with loving family and friends, keeps me moving forward, albeit very slowly!

My internal dialogue continues to be a critical aspect of managing the pain. I often remind myself that, as a therapist, I have never been better at what I do and continual learning and growing has been the key to constantly shifting my focus away from the pain. I fully realize and accept that by focusing and paying close attention to others' pain and using my knowledge and skills to be as helpful as I can be, I am able to postpone facing my own pain. I remind myself often of three motivational phrases:

1. What you focus on you make stronger.
2. Neurons that fire together wire together.
3. People will forget things you say but they will never forget how you made them feel.

It is steady and repetitive work, but this has become the foundation of my strategy for pushing through and giving me hope that I will get better and better at living my life more fully—despite the pain. Or perhaps I should say "along with the pain"?

It is important to speak about the therapeutic impact of having loving pets. From 1976 to the present day, we have been blessed with eight amazing Great Danes (Shayna, Skylar, Harleigh, Caesar, Charlotte, Stella, Maisie and Maggie) and one English bull terrier (Britty, a gift from friends). We fell in love with the Great Dane breed, even though their life span can be quite short. They have all been an active part of my coping strategies over the years, as I loved to lay with them, play with them and train them. For the most part, they were all well behaved, loving family members. I would often lay in bed with my ice packs, heating pad, etc., and cuddle with the puppies, which would get my oxytocin flowing! These loving companions have never betrayed my confidence, and always made me smile, laugh and cry. As painful as it is to lose such loving family members, I could never imagine my life without one!

I often talk with my clients about the therapeutic benefits of having pets. Having young people remember sitting or lying with their pet, stroking their coats, and feeling relaxed and calm is often "self-soothing." Focusing on specific sensations in the body (the feel of the fur on the fingers, the warmth, and the beating heart, for example) can be a powerful grounding technique—even a safe and quiet space to spend a few moments a day. When this becomes an easily retrievable memory, it can become a strategy for managing powerful emotions and pain.

Fortunately, my two sons are out on their own and making their way through life; they are trying to live out their dreams. Unfortunately, my strong right hand, the one person who has enabled me to function so well in so many ways—Annie—now makes me face what the true cost of all this has been to our relationship. To our life together.

Learning this has been a "foundational shift," like there was an earthquake and we have tried to figure out how and what we can rebuild. I hope I will be able to develop better control over this pain so I can give more personal attention to those I love the most: Annie, Ben and Luc, their partners (Rachael and Sarah) and our four amazing grandchildren (Rhyden, Finn, Sam and Milo). They provide the love and purpose that fuels my hope for the future.

All the time spent in bed, in agony, should have been time spent with Annie and the boys. I missed that time to play, to share, to enjoy each other's company. The most painful part of enduring chronic pain is that all that time is lost, gone forever. When I return, in my mind, to those long painful hours is bed, I imagine what my family may have been doing. I imagine the boys playing outside and wish I could have been there. I imagine Annie visiting with friends, sharing, laughing, and enjoying those relationships. I missed so much.

I also wish I was more helpful to Annie. The dogs had to be taken out and fed. Shopping had to be done, meals prepared, the house cleaned, conflicts between the boys resolved. Even though there were many times I would push myself to be present—to help as much as I could—I always felt it was not nearly enough. I remember times, lying in bed, struggling with the pain and trying to distract myself with the movies, guided meditations or music that played on my laptop while being aware of things happening downstairs. I could hear the boys talking, I could hear the doors open and close, I could hear Annie in the kitchen preparing a meal, and I could smell food cooking. During these moments, my pillow wet with tears, I so wished I was able to be with them—or just wished I wasn't around!

Once the sadness subsided, the anger would rise, and I would pound the pillows and scream into them. I knew that I needed to allow these emotions to breathe, however, the result was always increased pain in my head. Crying and getting angry consistently makes the pain worse. Following these episodes, I was always able to escape to one of my safe, quiet spaces. I imagined myself walking through the ravine on a warm sunny day or sitting on the rock at Cartwright Point, smelling the seaweed and the motor oil from the boats while the waves splashed against the rocks. Needing to sleep, I would reach for my medication and hope that I would be able to get some sleep and imagine swimming lengths in a pool.

When I spend time in bed trying to control the pain now, I am flooded with thoughts of all the things I should be doing as a partner, as a father and grandfather. But I have learned to accept these experiences and then shift away from them to the job of reducing the pain so I can be more involved as much as possible. Then the thought appears again: *I could live another twenty years like this! Fuck me!*

I continue to work at my social relationships. The most important aspect to feeling more connected with others is to stay mindful of my interest and caring for others and of what is happening in their lives. If you live with chronic pain, I expect this will resonate with you. It is so difficult to shift away from the pain, to leave it in the background so I can focus on others and fully enjoy the interactions. In the middle of conversation, a lightning bolt strikes behind my left eye that can distract me. It is easy to be distracted from interactions when the pounding in my temples increases or when out for a walk and my back pain acts up. It requires continued mindful practice to maintain meaningful and enjoyable relationships with others. This practice for me involves the continued development and implementation of daily rituals and routines.

I wrote out a schedule for a "routine" or "ritual" I wanted to engage in each morning that combined yoga, meditation (sitting and walking), positive imaging and chanting. Due to degenerative disc disease and spinal stenosis in my lower back, I had to, at the very least, do some stretches every morning so I could stand up straight (well, straight-ish) and walk properly. When the head pain is bad, these gentle exercises tend to make it worse for a while. I give myself a minimum of thirty minutes to engage in this ritual, which includes taking the dog for a walk, chanting and meditating, and I am convinced it pays off. When I chant, out loud or silently, I am in my "quiet space" where nothing else exists. The pain seems to be elsewhere in these few moments.

Another ritual I have used for years is not listening to anything when I am driving except for my own chanting and positive self-talk. This directs me to only pay attention to driving and not the throbbing/stabbing pain. I am easily distracted by the pain or the radio, so the chants and self-talk are automatic now, which allows me to remain alert and oriented to the task of driving.

Routines practiced frequently eventually become more automatic, making them a habit. From training in neurolinguistic programming, I learned that the vast majority of behaviours originate from positive intentions, however, sometimes there can be negative side effects that can create more problems. The positive intention behind taking more and more medication or changing medications has always been pain relief (physical and emotional). Once such behaviour becomes habitual, no other behaviour introduced as a replacement provides the same level of relief—initially—which is why it is so difficult to develop less harmful ways of achieving relief. The "bad habits" are always more effective because the intention to get immediate relief is more powerful than the intention to reduce self-harmful behaviour. However, in the long run, creating more positive habits is a healthier solution.

In my work I also use the chanting and positive self-talk to orient and focus myself on my patients, co-workers, and clients. Prior to every therapeutic session, I remind myself of the people I am about to connect with. I reiterate what their core struggles seem to be and that it is my intention to actively listen, validate, remain curious, explore, and hold off on assumptions and advice-giving until I have confirmed my understanding of their experiences. This ritual has also become more automatic.

There is no magic pill for anything, just as there is no one form of psychotherapy or counselling that works for everyone. There are a multitude of theories, and therapeutic techniques within each theory, that are aimed at helping individuals and families of all ages to change. For those seeking help, it is a quagmire of possible therapists and interventions. Not only do people struggle to figure out who they should contact but availability and cost often become insurmountable obstacles. This is a critical issue for those who live with chronic pain, as finances are so often an impediment to finding help. The majority of psychotherapists and counsellors abide by principles they have learned and adopted from different theories, and they utilize techniques from a broad range of therapeutic possibilities—even those who claim to be strictly one form or another. The successful counsellors are the ones with the ability to connect and present options to help their clients move towards the life they have always wanted. This is what informs my practice.

At this point in my career, each time I engage in therapeutic conversations with patients and clients, their stories trigger a range of images and metaphors that are often journey oriented. Swimming, canoeing, snorkelling, nature walks, hikes, climbs, gardening, flying, and so on come to mind and I am reminded that images and metaphors about our lives are limited only by the power of our imagination! I am increasingly encouraged about the power of our minds to change sensations throughout our bodies—temperature, tension, pain, heart rate, blood pressure, and emotions—after establishing a foundation of daily practice of diaphragmatic breathing. "Control" has never meant "stopping" emotions, negative or positive. Perhaps we should shift away from the terms "negative" and "positive," and instead talk about "difficult" and "enjoyable." Emotions often rise and recede like the ocean tide, and all emotions need to be accepted and experienced fully. It is important to work through the difficult emotions and fully embrace the "enjoyable" ones without trying to hold onto them. As we all know, they, too, pass! Chronic pain also rises and recedes even though the pain may never go away completely.

Chronic Pain: My Journey

To establish control over painful emotions, I must recognize when they are rising, understand and accept them without judgment, spend time with them so they settle, then shift my focus to other, more pleasant endeavours. I have long since shifted away from the experience of being upset and angry when the stabbing pain appears, as reacting that way only increases the pain. Acceptance and shifting my mind to my quiet space is the only strategy that keeps me from falling into that dark rabbit hole of helplessness and hopelessness. Maintaining a daily practice of acceptance and control have become a core aspect of my routines and rituals.

CHAPTER 9

CREATING SAFE QUIET SPACE

Every morning, thoughts like *I can't do this anymore, it's just too damn hard!* work their way into my awareness. Some days I struggle for hours to resurrect positive thoughts to resist the constant pain: *What you focus on, you make stronger. You are strong and you can get through this. The intensity of the pain constantly rises and falls.* I accomplish something every day despite the pull to give in. I have relentless empathy for others and myself. Accept, validate, move on!

Thankfully, my list of positive thoughts take up considerably more space than the troublesome thoughts, even though it has not always been so. Be that as it may, facing those first negative thoughts every morning (and the ones late at night) can still be all consuming. It will always be a hurdle I have to get over every day. There were far too many days in the past when I didn't get over that hurdle, choosing instead to numb everything and just watch others living on a screen. Watching movies and television shows has always been a positive distraction for me whenever the pain rose to that overwhelming point, but there is no sense of accomplishment in this practice.

Oh, such a sad state of affairs, you poor pain-ridden soul! There are so many other people in the world who live with more pain and suffering than you. Snap out of it and get moving! This thought sequence is my secret weapon. It keeps me engaged in my life as much as possible. Some days I have the troublesome thought that it may fail to do the job, and that scares me! Many parents use this strategy with their children, and it tends to backfire because it invalidates the feelings being experienced. When I explain this to parents, with their child present, they seem to understand and have an easier time grasping the importance of validation. However, with my adult rational mind, being aware that others live with more pain and anguish than I, remains an important reminder to keep going.

I work hard to stay inside that inner chamber of positive thoughts that has an invisible, protective shield I created, keeping the negative thoughts at bay. Engaging in the deep breathing and dropping into one of my own quiet spaces many times every day has, thankfully, become habitual. My subconscious mind is constantly working to keep me focused on being mindful of the present moment. A poem I recently wrote tried to capture this perspective.

Quiet Space

Every living creature, uniquely beautiful
Such is fact, not opinion
Recognizing and celebrating beauty in difference
Listening to the stories of others
Experience the essence of such stories
Pains and joys
Allows for clear understanding
And felt validation
The experience of the others.
Alone, a mountain to climb
Seems insurmountable

But together, with another
There is more hope
That climb becomes possible.
Longing for and dreading change
Holding onto the longing or giving in to the dread
No matter in the end, we all end up dead.
And when death is near, looking back,
Regrets piled up around us like bricks in walls
Moving, closing in, threatening to crush us
Existing within the mind's imagination.
Choose to imagine differently
Outside of that room, a space positively focused
A safe space from which to live fully
Mindful and accepting of all that comes
Our hearts and minds taking the lead
Making the most of what we have
Until it is time to move on.

This notion of a safe, quiet space inside each of us first came to me when I was around seventeen. My brother Brad and I were seated on our couch in the basement. Brad had his school textbooks laid out on the table in front of him, which became his makeshift "drum set." One text for the snare, two texts for the tom-toms, three texts for the kick drum and one thin text for the high-hat. He used real drumsticks and actually got good at playing "the books," so it was exciting to watch the eventual transition to an actual drum set! In any event, during this time period he was also demonstrating the art of meditation. During one session, I was trying to follow but was having difficulty keeping myself still. After a few moments Brad turned to me and said, "You have to find a calm, quiet space inside!" That phrase stuck with me and was the beginning of my motivation to create and develop my own safe space inside.

I meditated for as long as I could every day, but I soon realized that I just kept getting lost in my thoughts and didn't feel "grounded" at all. I started to meditate for brief periods when I would simply focus on what I was experiencing visually, auditorily and kinaesthetically immersed in the full extent of "now," so to speak. As I described earlier, I loved to sit in nature while meditating, and this time became essential. This calm, quiet space inside of me had always been there, and I could access it any time I wanted. So I did, many times every day. Gradually, this became my most potent grounding practice, allowing me to feel connected and balanced. Whether walking through the ravine, sitting by the creek or sitting on the rocks on the shore of the St. Lawrence River—all in my imagination—I was able to be still, calm and at peace. And the pain receded.

I was fortunate to find this path and would not be here if I had not. The more often I dropped into one of my safe spaces, I would see, hear, feel and smell new things. When that happens, the stronger and more available each space became. When I speak about this space getting "stronger," I am speaking about the speed with which that space can spread the "relaxed calm" throughout my body. I can feel the flow as it pushes all the stress and tension out, and my heart rate and blood pressure remain balanced and stable. As a result of my ongoing practice, I can feel this relaxed calm spread through my body and mind in a single, deep, slow breath (which usually lasts for thirty to forty seconds).

I often ask clients, patients and colleagues a central question: "When you have an important decision or choice to make in your life, is it better to do that from a place full of stress and anxiety or a place of relaxed calm?" Everyone always agrees—from a place of relaxed calm, obviously! However, it is easier said than done. A still, quiet, grounded and protected space exists in everyone. This space develops while the fetus is in the mother's womb and protects against the enormous stress and strain of the birthing process. Once out into the world, human infants continue to spend as much time within this space as they can—when they are sleeping, being held, cuddled, fed or just spending time gazing at the world around them. The infant gradually (or not so gradually) experiences the stress, strain and pain of daily living, which yanks them out of their safe space to face reality! That safe, quiet, and calm space doesn't go anywhere, but negative and stressful experiences within their environment can trigger anxiety and depression, which, in turn, can bury it. Anxiety (worries and fears) and depression (low motivation, sadness, helplessness and hopelessness) and the negative thoughts and feelings associated with them, can render the safe space unavailable.

We can access this space, strengthen it and make it more accessible, with diligent practice (and many people do). Anxiety and depression try to convince people that there is no such space or that spending time there is a waste. There are so many things you need to do, so sitting and doing nothing accomplishes nothing, etc. This way of thinking can become the major block to developing this quiet space inside. This is often the first obstacle that needs to be negotiated to experience the true value of such a practice. Troublesome thoughts aimed at stopping the quiet space practice simply come into our awareness, without invitation, and how we respond to their presence will determine their strength and whether they will succeed or not. Getting upset, arguing with them, or trying to ignore them tends to make them stronger. Accepting them as simply troublesome thoughts (*Ah ... just you again*) and returning to one's practice weakens them right away and they tend to fade and return a little less often.

Even after years of practice, repeating a quiet space guided meditation allows me to get some sleep at night. When pain wakes me, I repeat this process to return to sleep. Sometimes I'm successful for an hour or two, but I may also require additional pain medication. More often than not, I wake between 3:00 and 4:00 a.m. and the thoughts come automatically: *I can't do this anymore. Just let me sleep. Cancel everything.* Then, I continue to try and fall back to sleep and that never works! I am still trying to reason with myself that the time from when I wake to the time I actually get out of bed (around 5:00 or 5:30 on workdays) is wasted, a useless struggle and I would be far better off if I just got up when I awoke and began my morning routine. On days when I am not working, I often toss and turn in this struggle until 7:00, 8:00 or 9:00 a.m. This is also time wasted—more regrets to add to The Wall! It is my experience that the key to the effectiveness of the quiet space exercise is the frequent repetition, which sometimes feels boring. The destructive, annoying thought *This is such a waste of time, why bother!* pops up repeatedly, but I know the opposite is true. It is important and healthy use of my time!

For more than twelve years, I have refrained from using narcotics to reduce the pain. Jan has continuously reminded me that I should also dispense with the over the counter (OTC) analgesics—Tylenol, Advil, Aleve, Motrin, etc. He is convinced by the evidence that taking between three and six thousand milligrams of analgesics a day not only can make my pain worse, but it could also be interfering with the effectiveness of the migraine medications I have recently tried (140 mg of Aimovig injected once a month, which I took for 2 years at $1200 a month; and Zomig nasal spray or Eletriptan, which I could only use twice a week). I have struggled with this process of trying to eliminate or at least decrease my use of OTC analgesics, but I have continuously failed.

So, why do I continue to take the analgesics? In one of my many "aha" moments, I realized that the analgesics dropped the pain level by a few points but had also become a psychological need. I was doing everything I could to get the pain level to zero. Reaching for the pills seemed to settle my emotions and thoughts—particularly the imperative thought *Don't just lay here in pain you fucking idiot, take something!* So, I would, and this response became habitual.

My rational and wise minds have become stronger when it comes to pain management, and I believe this is the result of continued meditations, my feeble attempts to practice Bagua, Jan's constant encouragement, Annie's support and guidance, and reminding myself that I can actually get some enjoyment out of spending time with family and helping out more around the house. I could not recall a time when taking the analgesics was effective in reducing the pain by any more than a few points, however, many nights those few points make a difference and allow me to drift into sleep for a while. Spending time with others in a mindfully compassionate way helps enormously in leaving the pain in the background.

After almost forty years of living with this pain, I still held onto the goal of getting rid of it—trying everything I could to bring an end to the pain. I came to the realization that it is not going anywhere! I must accept this fact of my life and focus my attention on simply managing the pain, using other techniques (meditation, essential oils, hypnosis, exercise, and Bagua practice). I believe that the long practice of meditation and self-hypnosis has strengthened my subconscious mind so that it continually works behind (or underneath) my conscious awareness to keep me in as relaxed and calm a state as possible. This makes it possible to accept that there is always pain there and to do my best to ride out the more intense variety. I remind myself that the pain resolves and always returns to baseline.

As I write this now, the pain is sitting at an 8/10. It is a throbbing, pulsating blob sitting inside my forehead and behind my eyes. Trying to focus on what I am writing and how I can best put this all into words is difficult. Part of me wants to forget about it, to just let it all go, but another part of me seems determined to get it all down in a way that makes sense. At these times, I feel I am suffering with this pain, that it has a hold of my body and my mind. At the same time as I try to explain it, I want to escape it. I think back to the narcotics and how they initially dulled the pain completely and to the nerve blocks that erased the pain for ten to twelve hours. I yearn for that pain-free state.

I have two primary metaphors for the pain that resonate with my conscious and subconscious minds: the "ocean" and the "blue sky." The ocean represents the pain—always there, always some small waves—but as it intensifies, the waves grow significantly. When the pain is at 8/10, there are huge waves crashing into the rocks on the shore, but a sandy beach can be seen on a deserted island, so I imagine myself in a sailboat or on a surfboard riding the wave of pain as it moves towards the beach on this island. Eventually, the waves diminish, and we wash up on shore. The pain reduced, I can rest on the beach being mindful of the sights and sounds and feeling the warmth of the sun, sand, and the gentle breeze.

In the "sky metaphor" the sky represents my consciousness, my awareness, within my safe space. The sky is blue, the sun shining, and there are only a few small white clouds. Clouds represent the pain. As the pain builds, the sky darkens, storm clouds appear and thunder and lightning strike (always in my temples and behind my eyes). I remind myself that storms eventually pass, and I try to shift into one of my safe quiet spaces. On one occasion while riding out a storm, I wrote the following:

> My mind is not a physical structure somewhere in my brain. Like our soul, our mind exists wherever we choose it to be. My mind is an energy field made up of conscious and subconscious material. At a conscious level is my present awareness—what I see, hear, smell, taste, touch, imagine and what I think about these experiences. At the subconscious level of my mind, I can pull knowledge and memories of experiences in any of these "sense" areas into my awareness. Some memories, experiences and knowledge exist at a deeper subconscious level, which I don't have easy access to. This would include distant memories

and painful, traumatic experiences, which can be accessed using clear intention, motivation and inducing a "deep trance state" (through meditative practice and hypnosis).

My imagination plays a key role in understanding and establishing a clear sense of how my inner world operates. Sometimes when I am meditating, I imagine my mind (and my soul) similar to clouds that can float throughout my body, as in a "body scan," or actually merging with any aspect of my anatomy, including muscles, bones, organs, blood and immune system, for example. By imagining my mind floating to wherever I wish it to be, I can effect changes within my body. I can slow my heart, decrease my blood pressure, ease pain—all with intention, motivation and focus. The effective and efficient use of my mind is the primary key to my healing process, and this requires the daily practice of such routines.

It is my experience that access to any specific part of me is always through my mind, and connecting with my mind is always through my breath.

My conscious mind (that sky within my imagination) has several parts: a rational part, an emotional part, a physical part, a wise part, a spiritual part and an imaginative part.

My goal is always to seek integration and balance—to have all aspects of my mind understanding each other and working together to help me become the person I aspire to be. This person I aspire to be exists within my imagination. I can see the person I want to become. For me, this is most important if I truly hope to change and grow in that direction.

Having arrived at such understandings, I used to try, in vain, to hold onto calm, peaceful meditative states until I realized that accepting and appreciating such space "when I am in it" works out better than trying to hold onto it! It is always within such states of mind that I feel most in control and pain seems more manageable. There are times during meditation when I feel that integration of all aspects of me and my connection to the world at large. I liken these experiences to the Japanese Buddhist experience of "satori" (clear understanding) and the experience of "kensho" (my true nature). During such moments, which are fleeting, I experience a wave of peace and serenity wash over and through me. I desperately want to hold onto that experience, but the desperation to hold on just pushes it away. The more often I meditate, the more likely it is that I will have such experiences, and so I continue with my practice as often as possible.

Through my relationships with myself and family, in addition to my work with young people, adults and families, my belief system shifts constantly. I have come to understand that even our "core beliefs" shift and change (getting stronger, or weaker and open to revision) as a result of our interactions with others and the world at large. We are constantly searching for experiences that reinforce our core beliefs even though we often have experiences that put those beliefs into question, affecting our emotions and our thoughts. It is so helpful to remain in a position of being open to such changes, consistently moving us along the path to becoming a kinder and more compassionate being.

In those moments when I become aware of the pain, if I accept that the pain is there and shift my focus to something requiring my attention, the pain tends to weaken. Accepting that the pain is an unfortunate part of my life, I make my goal to always work towards limiting its negative impact on my life and the lives of those close to me. This is the mindset I continue to cultivate.

CHAPTER 10

EASIER SAID THAN DONE

This phrase may well be the one I repeat most often in my work. When I explain to patients and clients how to best use the wealth of therapeutic techniques available to us all, I always speak about my fundamental belief that the techniques that one chooses to use will be most helpful when you can make them automatic. Making a strategy automatic only happens through frequent repetition until it becomes a positive daily habit. This is usually the first time I will use that phrase, "I know this is easier said than done!" When I utter these words, people always nod. This notion of how much effort it takes to create and maintain positive habits clearly resonates with most people.

Next, we talk about how important it is to begin slowly. Take brief moments of practicing a particular skill you want to develop. Just a couple of minutes a day and repeated as often as it may come into your mind is a good place to start. This seems to make the task much less daunting and more enjoyable than trying to force oneself to practice for longer periods, which will come in time. In my clinical work, I use many different analogies to reinforce the notion that you are developing a specific skill so that you become expert at using it. It's just like learning to play a scale on an instrument, learning to ride a bike or skate, shoot a puck, kick a ball and so on.

"That makes sense," they say.

"It's easier said than done!" I say again.

I have always believed that I am responsible for myself. If there is something wrong in my life, then I am the one that must fix it. I have seen a variety of professionals: general practitioners, pain specialists, neurologists, psychologists, naturopaths, chiropractors, physiotherapists, psychotherapists and hypnotherapists and they were all helpful to some degree. However, I also spent long hours reading material on managing chronic migraines and chronic pain in general. As I want to keep this story about my experiences living with chronic pain, I am resisting the urge to shift to an academic and theoretical perspective. I will maintain the personal perspective and share the insights and renewed possibilities that grew out of my readings, investigations and practice.

I am fascinated with the mind and how it functions and struggles to establish control. The issue of control is a complex one that requires consideration of a variety of perspectives. From an illness perspective, I don't believe our minds can stop physical ailments from happening. Our mind can't stop a bone from breaking or a physical illness from occurring. Our mind can only respond, and that response clearly has an impact on the effectiveness of treatment and managing through the recovery process. From my perspective, my mind had no control over the infection I had in 1981 that led to the development of the headaches, but my mind responded to those events with a desperate search for relief—for an end to the pain. In the early stages, my mind struggled with anxiety, fear, frustration, anger and depression. There was a part of me that recognized the critical importance of establishing specific techniques for settling and training my mind to manage the chronic daily pain. There is an old Irish saying that always comes to mind: "What cannot be helped must be endured."

As mentioned before, I practiced meditation and mindfulness long before the onset of pain, which created a solid foundation on which I could build. My experiences with various forms of meditation have continued to be life altering and life sustaining, and they have formed what I believe to be the foundation of my beliefs about managing chronic pain. The trances that always occurred when meditating varied in depth but always left me feeling more in control of my thinking, my emotions, and the *pain*. I put "the pain" in italics to underscore a key principle from narrative therapy: *externalization*. This means thinking and speaking about unwelcome troubles as separate from who we are even though we experience such troubles inside our minds and bodies. So, in a nutshell, I think about "the" pain, not "my" pain. In my mind, this subtle difference in language places the pain outside of me, and it comes into my awareness to provide me with a troublesome experience I really do not want.

The same principle or technique can be applied to any trouble or problem. One can speak of "the" anxiety, "the" depression, "the" OCD, "the" eating disorder and so on. Life existed without the problem, and then the problem arrived and messed things up for us. The theory, as I understand it, is that if the problem is a part of who we are, it becomes more difficult to address it and to limit its negative influence on our lives. One could say it infiltrates the self, slowly infecting other aspects of self.

When I first started reading about neuroplasticity, I was intrigued by the notion that we can change the way our brains operate by training our minds. We can change the flow of neurochemicals in our brains. One of the core beliefs that has stuck with me to this day is *neurons that fire together, wire together*. The first time I read that statement, the thought of bad habits, phobias, obsessions and compulsions came to mind. It was an "aha" moment for me and significantly shifted the way I thought about any problem and the "coping mechanisms" people use to decrease the negative effects on their lives. I had already learned through diaphragmatic breathing and meditating that I could lower my heart rate and blood pressure and create a powerful sensation of peaceful calm throughout. But I also realized I had changed the way neurochemicals flow in my brain because I had made a positive, daily habit of the deep breathing and meditation.

Holy shit! As mentioned before, one of the most troublesome yet most common thoughts when meditating was (and still is) *This is such a waste of time. You have so many more important things to do than just sit here and do nothing!* It turns out that meditating could be the most important thing we can do for our physical and mental health!

I read a story about a middle-aged man in California who suffered from chronic, debilitating sciatica. The pain would shoot down both legs and make it impossible for him to walk without the pain. He began sitting meditations and focused his mind on his lower back—all the muscles, tendons and nerves. In time he developed an image of the workings of his lower back and found that when he focused his attention on that area, he could decrease the pain. Then he began walking meditations during which he would focus his "trance state" on his lower back in his mind, soothing the nerves, muscles and tendons. The pain decreased as he engaged in walking meditation, so he increased the distance he walked. He found that when he would get distracted, he would experience an increase in the pain. Eventually he was able to take long walks without the debilitating pain shooting into his legs as long as he maintained his mindful focus.

Although one can find anecdotal stories in the literature to support almost anything, this story resonated with me, and I incorporated this focus on the muscles, tendons, membranes, and nerves in my head and aimed mental energy at soothing the painful areas. I relaxed the muscles in the neck and the tiny muscles in my head and face and then imagined inflamed nerves settling. This practice has become part of my daily rituals when meditating before work and before a session with a patient or client. Relax the body, focus the mind, reduce the swelling in the membranes, ease the tension in the tiny muscles and capillaries … and the pain eases.

In 2014, I increasingly experienced lower back pain (degenerative disc disease and spinal stenosis were diagnosed)

Chronic Pain: My Journey

and arthritis beginning in joints in my fingers and hands. I am presently working to include these muscles and joints in my daily practice. Once again, it rests on my ability to search and locate the space in my mind that can numb the pain, which requires significant collaboration with my subconscious mind through self-hypnosis and trance work. Through a typical induction process, listening to a guided meditation or simply using self-talk, I drop into a quiet space of mine, connect with my observing self and my subconscious mind (which I see as attached to my safe quiet spaces), and begin the process of shifting the sensations throughout my extremities. The fingers, hands, toes and feet have always been the best places to focus on changing sensations. The theory is that if I can change the sensation of warmth in my fingers to cold and then to numb, I can create that experience anywhere in my body.

So, when I sit, breathe and focus, I am able to experience some numbness in my hands, back and head, which reduces the pain level. However, when I change my focus to the here and now and whatever I need to do—whether that is take Maggie for a walk, have a conversation with someone, read or write—the pain returns. Sometimes the process is more effective than other times because there are so many independent variables that affect both the pain and my ability to focus my mind. This makes it difficult to predict when such strategies will be effective. However, the few moments I spend following my breath down into a quiet space, shifting my attention to the patient or client I am about to meet with, and opening myself to that experience has become a positive habit that continues to pay off.

When I begin a therapeutic session, I am fully present and open to whatever the person wishes to share. When the pain is at a level that interferes in the preparation process, I reach for the medications to try and drop the pain level, even just by a couple of notches. Having tried the various triptans, I have found that the Zomig nasal spray and Axert are the most effective for me. I also use the OTC medications: Tylenol, Motrin, Aleve, Robaxacet.

I alternate and at times combine. When I am off work, I am able to use a 1:1 balanced medical cannabis oil (<10% THC & >20% CBD) that can drop the pain level a couple of notches and improve my mood and sociability, which allows me to get more enjoyment from my important relationships. I must admit that when I remember the first few months I was taking the narcotics and they significantly numbed the pain, I yearn to be pain free. But I know the consequences of going down that path are dark and destructive in every way.

It is our mind's infrastructure that will determine our mental—and to a great extent our physical—health. I have witnessed it over many years of treating young people who have somatoform and conversion disorders. Our minds can collect all the emotional and psychological pain and converting that into physical symptoms that significantly reduce the level of emotional pain—the conversion becoming ego-syntonic. There is little or no anxiety in the person regarding the physical symptom(s). It is often easier in the short run for family to be supportive of a member who has physical symptoms where the "problem" is obvious. When someone has a problem that is not so obvious, as with chronic pain conditions, it is easy for others to "forget" that this person lives with the daily experience of pain. There is a stigma attached to such "invisible problems." Humans are skilled at hiding that which is not obvious, so the people in our lives have a hard time understanding what's going on.

As mentioned previously, I attended many workshops in narrative practice through the '80s and '90s (with Michael White), and then I trained and was eventually certified in narrative therapy in 2004. There are so many principles that have become anchors for me in my clinical practice and in my daily struggles with pain. One such principle involves "landscapes" within our mind—a landscape of identity, a landscape of action, a landscape of emotion, a landscape of cognition, a landscape of our primary relationships and so on. I imagine that connecting with each of these landscapes appear like a "drop-down" box where various aspects of that landscape appear. Through the lenses of my "observing self," I can change any aspect of each landscape to facilitate movement in a positive, adaptive direction.

Considering my mind as a variety of such landscapes has been helpful to me in separating the landscape of pain from all the others, which reduces the pain's impact on other areas. During my training in hypnotherapy, I spent considerable time trying to determine how to engage my subconscious mind in revamping some of those landscapes. Within the landscape of pain, I now have three primary areas: head pain (migraines), back pain (stenosis/arthritis) and hand pain (arthritis) including a variety of pain qualities (mild, moderate, severe, stabbing, throbbing and so on). In my "mapping" practice aimed at restructuring the landscape of pain, I imagine my primary safe space on the shores of the St. Lawrence. I am sitting on the rocks by the beach on Cartwright Point, and the waves on the river represent the pain. Some waves represent the migraines, others the back pain or arthritis in my hands. Some waves rise into whitecaps, curling into themselves as they roll towards shore while others may crash against the rocks below me. Sometimes I see dark storm clouds, wind, and lightning. Through my breath, into my trance, I can part the clouds, bring out the sun, calm the river's waves and enjoy the peacefulness of this space. The pain weakens in response. I have also found myself dropping into my safe quiet space at my centre without the full visualization of a specific place. This allows me to quickly become relaxed, calm and focused within two deep, slow breaths.

Over the past year, I have been dropping into this space more often, sometimes a few times a day. Whatever situation I am heading into, I continue to ask my favourite questions: *What is your intention here?* Answering this question helps me to remain relaxed, calm and mindful. This process happens in less than two minutes, however, at times when the pain is too intense to focus, I reach for the medications to help reduce the intensity.

I try to remain hopeful that this practice will continue to have a positive and cumulative effect on my general pain level and how I manage it. There is little doubt in my mind that the years of daily meditation using diaphragmatic breathing have become the foundation of my pain management protocol and to a large extent have become automatic.

In the landscape of my mind, I remain convinced of the correlation between the characteristics of my pain and the changes in temperature of more than ten degrees within a twenty-four-hour period, humidity and pressure (particularly storms). In addition, simply shifting into another season negatively impacts the pain, however, climate change seems to have complicated so many physical ailments, such as allergies, arthritis, and the continuum of pain disorders. So many folks I talk to who have seasonal allergies attest to their experience of symptoms that are now year-round! As individuals we have no control over climate changes or the weather. We can only establish some control over how we respond to the changes in our physical, psychological, and emotional experiences.

I have recently reconnected with my innate love of swimming and found that the time I spend in the pool is close to pain free in my lower back in particular, but also in my head. The moment I enter the pool, I enter a trance state within the landscape of my mind. My body automatically starts the breaststroke, my cupped hands reaching out in front of me, pulling the water to my sides as my legs frog kick. Of all the strokes I learned, the breaststroke was always my favourite. Focusing on the sensations in my body as the water moves around me has become a powerfully grounding experience. I am mindful of the warm water, the aroma of chlorine, the softness of the water as my arms and legs gently push and pull the water during each length of the pool. On my way home from each swim, I find myself thinking that if I can achieve that level of a meditative trance state in the water, this will increase the power of this quiet space so I can drop-in and enjoy that level of relief! This remains a work in progress.

The whole quiet space practice continues to reinforce itself in so many ways. When sitting in meditation and noticing what comes up in body and mind, various metaphors frequently come to mind. One of the more recent metaphors is around the "structure of the mind." Like all structures that need to withstand all sorts of weather, a strong, solid foundation is critical. Creating a solid, strong foundation is simple, but it takes care and patience to build before you can safely add all the other parts. I have come to view the foundation of my mind as the quiet space—grounded, calm, relaxed and focused. From here I can add, change, renovate any part of how my mind operates in the landscape of pain. Without such a strong foundation, this structure would surely collapse!

Our bodies begin to break down as we age, which is a widely understood and accepted part of life. I understand that the amount of pain and suffering that accompanies this process is primarily determined by one's physical and mental health. In December 2021, I had consulted with Jan about the severe pain travelling down my legs. This resulted in another MRI and appointments with a neurophysiologist who had a machine that sent an electrical current through various places on my legs. Then I went to see a neurosurgeon who interpreted all the data and suggested a surgical procedure—a laminectomy—which was carried out in February 2022.

The results are mixed! There was no more pain down my left leg but there remained intermittent pain down the front of my right leg. This made it difficult to walk more than half a block without it feeling like a blow torch sending the fire down my right thigh to my knee. This made work at the hospital difficult because of the pain. It would come on after standing for more than five minutes in one position or when walking more than five hundred metres. When it came, it was impossible to continue, and

I had to sit and lift my right leg across my left knee. After about five minutes the pain subsided, and I could carry on for a while. Consequently, I have only been working eight-hour shifts at the hospital instead of the long twelve-hour shifts I did for so many years. Even the eight-hour shifts can be a struggle.

I had a follow-up appointment with the neurosurgeon a month following the surgery, and he explained that we needed to give it more time to see if the pain in my right leg would settle on its own. The fact that the sciatica down my left leg was gone gave us some hope. The surgery may have been traumatic for the femoral nerve on the right side, so if the pain persists, we will need to repeat the whole process again to establish where that nerve is having trouble.

In the meantime, I continue with some success in imagining applying ice to that nerve and experiencing the cold sensation in the thigh and a reduction in the pain. Sometimes it works and sometimes it doesn't! When I am walking, I imagine that nerve in my mind's eye being free floating, as if floating in water, with nothing pressing on it or interfering in any way. Then I add ice to the water and the nerve becomes numb. Again, sometimes this is helpful and other times not so much! The Lyrica my doctor prescribed was not helpful, and after a month at maximum dosage, we switched to 120 mg of Cymbalta. It provided relief in both my back and leg, which is a significant success!

In spite of the strategies I use on a daily basis to stay present, in the here and now without getting pulled into the pool of pain, it remains a struggle to get moving every day. The positive self-talk is so important first thing in the morning, as it sets the stage for moving in that direction.

When you live with chronic daily pain, everything is experienced through the pain. When sitting, standing or walking, or even eating, the pull is always to the area in the body experiencing the most pain in that moment. I just pushed myself to take my daily walk past beautiful old trees, amazing homes, kids playing, rain falling gently, a variety of stores with smells of baking, folks walking their dogs. And the entire time, I tried to remain mindful of all that I was seeing, hearing and smelling instead of that nagging pain in my back, my leg and my head. Avoiding that pull into the pain takes daily practice of both the mind and the body, and continuing this daily practice so often requires a significant physical, emotional and psychological push. Most of the time, if I am being honest with myself, I don't "feel like" walking, playing music or swimming. I feel like crawling back into bed and being still with an ice pack on my head. But when I push myself to engage in those activities, I find that I get some enjoyment out of them, and when I look back on the day, I feel proud that I did it. I have not found a way to constantly numb the pain, but every strategy I use—medication, meditating, self-hypnosis, music and exercise—is an essential component of my regimen that keeps me getting up each morning and moving through each day one day at a time!

As mentioned, from within any safe, quiet space, I often connect with my observing self and look at how my experience of pain has impacted every area of my life, including the development of this manuscript. I have spent significant time writing so many times only to become lost and frustrated, deleting what I just wrote, closing the file and not returning to it for weeks or months. The pain often intensifies as I struggle to find a good "flow"—a clear writing "zone". It feels choppy and tangential and then the negative thoughts creep in: *This is never going to flow ... You are not a writer ... Editors will just laugh and think you're joking ... No way this will ever reach publication ... You may as well pack it in now!*

Lately, when the throbbing has been steady, several bones in my face and head become painful to touch. The bones on the sides of my forehead, under my eyebrows, and just below my eyes hurt. This pain can last for hours or days and makes massaging my head and face more painful. However, the ice packs provide some temporary relief. The stabbing pain that occurs behind my eyes (I think of these as lightning strikes), usually behind one eye at a time, thankfully only occur two or three times a week when the migraine pain peaks at about 9/10. Each "strike" lasts between sixty seconds and five minutes, and I will most often take my migraine medication when the first strike occurs. Although the strikes often continue intermittently for about an hour, I believe that the medication prevents this experience from lasting longer. Years ago, I experienced similar pain in the bones and behind my eyes, but it became less often. During my recent fifteen-day experience with the COVID-19 virus, this intensity of head pain became a daily experience again. Now two months after the virus passed, this pain continues daily, requiring the application of ice packs two to three times a day.

Through a variety of readings in neuroscience, I have come to appreciate that our physical brain does not actually distinguish the "real" from the "imagined." If I take a few moments to imagine that I have fallen into a pit of snakes (one of my nightmares as a child), I can feel the adrenaline flow. My fight/flight response in my amygdala has been activated even though I am not actually in a pit of snakes. This is true for other phobias as well, which is why exposure therapy can occur through hypnosis. At times when I am with friends, out for dinner or in sessions with clients when it is not appropriate to put an ice pack on my head, I imagine the cold ice around my head and at least feel some relief.

Our imagination plays a key role in our lives in ways we often forget. For example, if I want to get along better with someone, I have to be able to imagine that difference to actually make those changes. It is important to see how I would behave differently and how the other person would respond. If I cannot see the change, it will not happen.

The effectiveness of hypnotherapy depends on our clients' ability to access and use their imagination to experience a variety of bodily sensations and to consider the ways they would like to change to become the person they aspire to be. If I wish to stop being so angry at other drivers on the road, I have to see myself, in my imagination, responding differently. I must remind myself that there could be several unknown reasons a driver is driving poorly, so my job is to remain relaxed, calm and focused on my driving.

Those of us who live with chronic daily pain are fully aware of the impact it has on us and our loved ones physically, emotionally, psychologically, and spiritually. When the pain arrived, relationships changed dramatically and continued to change in ways we never dreamed of—and certainly never hoped for. This struggle continues day by day, hour by hour, minute by minute, and I try to feel grateful for any amount of time that I can enjoy moments of reduced pain.

And so, I keep going … as best I can.

CHAPTER 11
SEMI-RETIREMENT

As I approach seventy-two years of age, I have decided to retire from my job at SickKids, which will give me two open days a week. I will likely add one day to my private practice, so I have three days seeing private clients. The other day I am hoping to volunteer in some form working with horses or other animals, perhaps at the humane society. I have a deep love of animals (other than snakes and squirrels!) that started with a donkey ride when I was about five. I loved spending time with my grandparents' dog Boots in Kingston, our own dogs, and spending a summer at Barb and Elton's farmhouse with their horse Mica.

I have always had a love for and fascination with horses and would welcome an opportunity to engage in some way with equine therapy. The literature on equine therapy says that being with and caring for horses can have several positive effects on children and adults who struggle with mental health issues and have poor self-esteem. Simply being in the presence of such majestic creatures apparently decreases the flow of the stress hormone cortisol and increases the flow of oxytocin, which has a calming effect on our body and mind. It has been said that horses are emotionally sensitive and can tell if someone is upset, angry, afraid, or sad. Anyone who lives with dogs and cats will likely say the same of them.

There is a part of me that is very much looking forward to this next chapter in my life and another part of me that worries about the trajectory of the pain that accompanies me. *Will it get any better or will it get worse?* This is the upsetting fear that impacts every person who lives with pain, but it is crucial to avoid getting caught in that cycle of negative thought and emotion. I have no control over the future, so I can only use the skills I have developed to cope with whatever pain I may have. Jan continues to share his belief that, at the very least, some of the pain is the result of analgesic overuse, and he continues to encourage me to go off them for two to three months to see how it impacts the pain frequency and intensity. This would likely mean many weeks of increased pain using only a combination of pressure (tight head bands) and ice packs applied to forehead and temples. I have not yet been able to psyche myself up for that!

Alan Gordon's book *The Way Out* (2021) has added to my understanding of pain. He speaks about the difference between "structural pain" and "neuroplastic pain." Maybe some of the pain I experience is the result of damage to membranes and nerves in my head from repeated infections and the early head injury (structural pain), but there is significant intensifying of the pain due to habitual impact of anxiety, fear, and depression (neuroplastic pain). So my understanding of my experience of the pain is that my brain responds to the chronic pain as "danger," and increases the flow of cortisol (the stress hormone), triggering anxiety and fear. This increases the intensity of the pain, which can merge with feelings and thoughts of helplessness and hopelessness. Through my daily practice of meditation, I can now more easily ease that anxiety and fear, which decreases the intensity of the pain. Even just a point or two makes a difference in my mood because I feel like I have a little more control, and it helps me manage my daily activities.

I hope those of you who live with chronic pain have found that some of my experiences and understandings resonate with you. Once again, it is not my place to advise the reader but perhaps you've even found a few new techniques for pain management that you can speak with your professional team about. So much of this ongoing practice involves trial and error; we try new things to see how they work or don't work. My experiences have consistently established and reinforced the need for multiple tools that are practiced daily. I also aim to develop new, positive daily habits, the foundation of which is always the diaphragmatic breathing.

I have conceptualized the mindset that I have been developing for years as a material structure in "The Positive Structure of the Mind" (manuscript in process). I imagine this as how a house is built. A solid foundation to the house is critical, and the same is true for the mind. The foundation of a positive mind is the development of an expertise in the use of diaphragmatic breathing. This form of deep breathing that is thousands of years old can become a daily automatic practice, with the help of the subconscious, to maintain one's quiet and protected space inside.

The basement level above the foundation, in my mind's house, is composed of four "core" beliefs: that all life is sacred; our environment is precious and must be cared for; humans are born primarily altruistic; and love and compassion are stronger than hate and prejudice.

The first floor is comprised of acceptance and compassion for self and others where the daily practice of diaphragmatic breathing becomes the breath of love. Spending the beginning of each day on this first floor sets the stage for a mindful and productive day and avoids the slip into judgment and prejudice.

The second floor, although it is an open space concept, has specific areas of functioning which capture the four virtues of Bagua: honesty with self and others (gentle transparency); humility in thought, word and deed; service to others according to their needs (helping kindness); and sincerity, the foundation of every action.

The third floor of my mind's house, also open space, has three primary areas of mind: my emotional mind; my rational mind; and my wise mind. All require care, so they grow to full capacity.

The breath of love (the diaphragmatic breathing) flows through the mind's house and is essential for the growth, integration, and balance within the mind.

Now, a mind well-built structurally and enhanced daily can withstand emotional storms or destructive, thought-filled whirlwinds without severe damage. When experiences are joyful, we can enjoy them fully, mindfully, without a need to hold onto them. When experiences are emotionally or physically painful, I can drop down to the basement, connect with my quiet and protected space through my breath and move through the pain as best I can. All important decisions and choices in life ought to be made from this space that involves our emotional, rational and wise minds.

My daily practice involves a few minutes of practice, every morning and every night of diaphragmatic breathing. I drop down into that quiet space and accept the pain at whatever level of intensity it is at, which eases the fear that always accompanies it. That fear must also be accepted as understandable, but to focus one's attention on it, makes it increasingly stronger. I then shift my focus to either preparing for my day in the morning or for my sleep at night. Following the morning ritual, I try to practice gentle stretching and the Daoyin of Jiulong Baguazhang. This ritual practice keeps the structure of my mind's "house" strong and sustainable and, along with the medications, helps me to feel more grounded and balanced. Pain is always, unfortunately, along for the ride, and there is no way of knowing how it may shift in the future - my fear is that it will get worse, my hope is that it will get better! I choose to work at staying busy and focusing on hope.

ACKNOWLEDGEMENTS

I would like to express my sincere thanks to; Rob Chatwin and David Avery who reviewed an early draft of the manuscript and provided support for moving forward and Jan Castoniu, who provided continuous, compassionate support over more than twenty years. Thank you to Brad for introducing me to the power of meditation.

Thank you also to Judi and Chaim for their counsel and all our close friends who have been so understanding, supportive and loving, throughout this journey. Thank you to Penny, who encouraged me to write my story.

Thank you to my publishing team at Tellwell. Thank you to Annie, my best friend, and the love of my life, for being with me through this ordeal.

BIBLIOGRAPHY

Baddeley, Alan (2004) *Your Memory – A User's Guide*, Firefly Books Ltd.
Brazier, David (1995) *Zen Therapy*, John Wiley and Sons Inc.
Brown, Brene (2015) *Rising Strong*, Spiegel & Grau
Brown, Brene (2021) *Atlas of the Heart*, Random House
Chodron, Thubten (2004) *Taming of the Mind*, Snow Lion Publications
Cleaver, Eldridge (1968) *Soul On Ice*, McGraw-Hill
Csikszentmihalyi, Mihaly (1990) *flow*, Harper & Row
Daitch, Carolyn (2007) *Affect Regulation Toolbox*, W. W. Norton & Company
Denborough, David (2014) *Retelling the Stories of Our Lives*, W. W. Norton & Co.
Doidge, Norman (2015) *The Brain's Way of Healing*, Viking Penguin
Donoghue, Paul J.; Siegel, Mary (1992) *Living with Invisible Chronic Pain*, Norton
Epstein, Mark (2022) *The Zen of Therapy*, Penguin Press
Fox, Michael J. (2009) *Always Looking Up*, Harper Collins
Frewen, Paul; Lanius, Ruth (2015) *Healing the Traumatized Self*, W. W. Norton & Co.
Gilbert, Paul (2018) *Living Like Crazy*, Annwyn House
Goldstein, Elisha (2012) *The Now Effect*, Simon $ Schuster Inc.
Gordon, Alan (2022) *The Way Out*, Avery Publisher

Grant, Mark (2016) *Change Your Brain-Change Your Pain*, BookPOD

Hunter, D.; Webster, C.; Konstantareas, M. & Sloman, L. (1982). Children in Day Treatment: A Child Care Follow-up study. *J of C&YC, 1*;1 45-58

Hunter, D.S. (1983) Nicola: The use of sign language with a blind, autistic child. *Child & Youth Care Forum, 47* 12: 321-336.

Hunter, D.S. and Webster, C. D.(1984). Children in day treatment: A four to eight year follow up. *J of C&YC, 2*;1 27-40

Hunter, Don, S., (June 1989) The use of physical restraint in managing out-of-control behavior in youth: A frontline perspective *Child & Youth Care Forum, 53* 18(2): 141-154

Hunter, Don S. and Armstrong, Harvey (1994). Establishing Group Supervision Within a Group Psychotherapy Program. *J of C&YC, 9*;4 51-62.

Hunter, Don S. (1995). The Association Between Psychiatric Admission and Birthdays Among Inpatient Adolescents. *J of C&YC, 10*;1 43-55.

Hunter, Don S. (2022) Website Blog. *donshunter.org* A Balanced Life: Living with Chronic Pain

Jinpa, Thupten (2015) *A Fearless Heart*, Penguin Press

Kapleau, Philip (1980) *The Three Pillars of Zen*, Anchor Books

Kessler, David (2019) *Finding Meaning*, Scribner Books

Li, Cynthia (2019) *Brave New Medicine*, Reveal Press

Meichenbaum, Donald (1974) Self Instructional Strategy Training, *Human Development, 17*: 273-280

Moore, Thomas (1992) *Care of the Soul*, Harper Collins

Moore, Thomas (2014) *A Religion of One's Own*, Penguin Random House

Schwartz, Richard (2021) *No Bad Parts*, Sounds True Publishing

Thomelin, Zetta (2018) *The Healing Metaphor*, Grosvenor House Publishing

Tirch, Dennis (2012) *Overcoming Anxiety*, New Harbinger Publications

Webster, Jamieson (2019) *Conversion Disorder*, Columbia University Press

White, Michael; Epston, David (1990) *Narrative Means to Therapeutic Ends*, Dulwich Centre

Wiest, Brianna (2020) *The Mountain is You*, Thought Catalogue Books, NY

Yapko, Michael (2021) *Process-Oriented Hypnosis*, W. W. Norton & Co.

APPENDIX A

Jiulong Baguazhang
(Bagua)

The Daoyin
1. Neck Rotations
2. Push the Sky
3. Press Heaven and Earth
4. Draw the Bow
5. Leaning Temple
6. Dragon Looks Around
7. Square Stepping
8. Cobra Descends from the Moon
9. Dragon Serves Tea
10. The 5 Circles (over, under, across, up, down)
11. Clearing (Qui Gong)

ABOUT THE AUTHOR

Don is a psychotherapist who has been educated and trained in a broad range of therapeutic modalities, including psychodynamic, client-centred, cognitive, solution-focused, narrative, emotion-focused, hypnosis, neurolinguistic programing, eye movement desensitization and reprocessing, compassion-focused, and mindfulness therapies. He has extensive experience in hospitals, community mental health clinics and private practice, providing counselling to children, youth, adults, couples and families. Don was also a part-time professor in child and youth counsellor programs at colleges and university for over ten years. Retiring in December 2022 from the hospital scene, Don is continuing with his private practice in Toronto, Ontario, Canada.

Manufactured by Amazon.ca
Bolton, ON